Blood: The Science, History, and Mysteries of Life's Vital Flow

Guglielmo Mariani • Peter M Lydyard
Pier Mannuccio Mannucci

Blood: The Science, History, and Mysteries of Life's Vital Flow

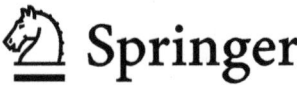 Springer

Guglielmo Mariani
Department of Haematology
University of L'Aquila Medical School
(Retired)
Roma, Italy

Peter M Lydyard
Division of Infection and Immunity
University College of London
London, UK

Pier Mannuccio Mannucci
Centro Emofilia e Trombosi Angelo
Bianchi Bonomi
Fondazione IRCCS Ca' Granda Ospedale
Maggiore Policlinico
Milan, Italy

ISBN 978-3-031-92480-4   ISBN 978-3-031-92481-1   (eBook)
https://doi.org/10.1007/978-3-031-92481-1

Cover Image: Prof. Guglielmo Mariani. High resolution image of red blood cells

This Springer imprint is published by the registered company Springer Nature Switzerland AG
The registered company address is: Gewerbestrasse 11, 6330 Cham, Switzerland

If disposing of this product, please recycle the paper.

Foreword

The Authors have written this book because of their longstanding interest in blood, a science they have taught and conducted research on, producing significant clinical and scientific contributions to the diagnosis of blood, immune disorders, and patient management. This work has been designed to be as clear and comprehensible as possible to a diverse group of individuals who are interested in blood and its multiple meanings and functions. Further, a glossary is provided at the end of the text because several technical terms may not be familiar to the readers. Note that words with an * the first time they appear in the text are explained in the Glossary where terms are listed alphabetically.

Prof. of Haematology Universities of Rome,   Guglielmo Mariani
L'Aquila and Palermo (retired) Rome, Italy
Visiting Professor University of Westminster London
(2014–2020), London, UK

Emeritus Professor, University College London   Peter M Lydyard
London, UK
Visiting Professor/Researcher, University of Westminster,
London, UK
Associated Professor, University of Georgia
Tbilisi, Georgia

Emeritus Professor, University of Milan   Pier Mannuccio Mannucci
and Research Fellow, Fondazione IRCCS Ca'
Granda Ospedale Maggiore Policlinico, Milan, Italy

About the Book

This book is about the discovery of blood, the tools that have been developed for the identification of blood components, and how blood components are now used in the treatment of a wide range of serious diseases. All living beings need blood, but there are intrinsic differences among species that evolved through genetic changes caused by different living environments. Blood provides nutrients and oxygen to tissues and organs and removes impurities by carrying them to specialized organs such as the kidneys. Other specialized organs, the lymph nodes, the spleen, and the liver, remove abnormal/diseased cells. Furthermore, blood participates in most of the defense mechanisms of our body and plays a crucial role in maintaining the balance of the body's systems carrying hormones and other chemical messengers.

The authors describe some iconic diseases (anemia, hemophilia, thrombosis) that are relevant to understanding how blood disorders occur and manifest themselves. They also discuss novel therapies (target, cellular, and immune therapies) for some of the most severe blood diseases, illustrating the incredible scientific progress that has occurred in the past few decades.

Introduction

Every day, millions of people have diagnostic laboratory tests or donate blood. Why is blood so important? Blood reaches every remote corner of our being, provides nutrients, carries oxygen, and removes impurities from tissues. Blood is not only a transport and defense system, but it also plays a crucial role in maintaining the balance of all the other body systems. All living beings (whether they are warm-blooded, such as mammals and birds, or cold-blooded, as insects, reptiles, amphibians, and invertebrate animals) live thanks to blood, which is essential for life. We all take its existence and importance for granted, without knowing what it contains and its countless and amazing properties.

The word blood, in French "sang," in German "blut," in Italian "sangue," in Spanish "sangre," derives from the Indo-European languages where "sak" means flow: in archaic Latin it became "sanguen" and then sanguis. The Greek word "aima" means heat or "make red" or "make warm" and from it the term Hematology was derived: the science studying blood. The English term blood (blöd in old English) derives from the German blut.

This book is a voyage we would like to take with our readers: it is organized into four parts, going from the history of blood, its relation with religion in ancient populations, through the basic science of blood to its disorders and its use in treating a variety of diseases. The study of blood, from a historical perspective, has given rise to the many branches of specialized medicine as we know them today.

Contents

Part III Disorders of the Blood

Part IV Blood and Disease Management

Part I
History

Chapter 1
Religious and Social Aspects

Religious Aspects

In some ancient and primitive religions, a sacrifice with blood was thought to be appreciated by the Gods and was considered a supreme gift to appease them. The sacrifice of animals is still performed in some populations.

The Bible frequently mentions blood and identifies it with life itself: 'the life of the flesh is in the blood'. Blood is considered so holy that in the Old Testament, the Divine Law forbids its consumption. This is the reason why Jehovah's Witnesses, who interpret the Bible in the strict sense, refuse blood transfusions. The Jewish religion does not forbid meat as a food (except the hare, the camel, and pig), but animal meat during preparation needs to be deprived of blood, so it becomes "kosher" (food that is made pure). The prescriptions of the Koran for Muslims are very similar: pork cannot be eaten, and animals when need to be butchered must be deprived of their blood. Traditionally, the catholic religion gives great symbolic importance to blood with the 'blood of Jesus Christ', which even represents a sacrament.

Blood in Ancient Civilizations

For the Egyptians, blood was the vehicle of life and to appease Shesmu, the God of blood, a vindictive God, they offered wine as a symbol of blood. In Homer's poems, blood is the expression of a tribal, familiar, patriotic bond, and the knowledge that the features related to it were 'transmitted' to descendants was considered an important value. For Hippocrates, the four body humors were: yellow bile, black bile, mucus (or phlegm), and blood. For Herodotus 'the members of a family have the same blood' and the braves have 'good and virtuous blood'. In Ancient Greece, blood was identified with the psyche, but later the physical concept that 'blood is a warm fluid through which the animal is nourished' became established. Galen identified two types of blood, the 'dark' (venous), which he thought stemmed from the liver after food 'conversion', and the 'red one' that originated from the heart. In Chinese medicine, blood is a vital substance that is inseparable from the vital energy (Qi), of which it represents the physical form. Blood gives rise to Qi through the nutrition of tissues.

The Beginnings of a Scientific Approach to Understanding Blood

In essence, blood has been recognized as a fundamental body constituent by all ancient cultures, indistinguishable from life and, at times from the character of the individual. For more than a thousand years, this philosophers' and classical doctors' interpretation remained unquestionable, it was a kind of dogma, to which the Christian Churches abided.

Medical science, therefore, did not make substantial progress until the Renaissance, when art and science underwent the revolution we today call 'Humanism'. This opened the door to observation of natural phenomena with a new eye, a curious one. Nature was observed and admired for how it has produced plants and animals, in a way where 'nothing is lacking and nothing is superfluous', as Leonardo Da Vinci said. It is thanks to the immense curiosity of Leonardo that observation of Nature became science. Man changed his vision with Humanism and Leonardo, for the first time, tried to interpret the functioning of the various organs and systems with a mechanistic approach. He postulated that muscles and tendons have postural functions and, through the joints, a system of levers and counter-levers is actioned. Another innovative approach of Leonardo was the mechanics of fluids (hydraulics): he discovered the way that blood flows and was the first to hypothesize that blood took a 'circular' route. From this concept derives the term 'circulation'.

However, Leonardo had too many ongoing interests, he was taking notes of everything he observed or that came into his mind. These observations were sketched in his notebook, which he always kept hanging from his waist. Therefore, he rarely managed to finish a study but accomplished it only years later. Those of his contemporaries who were less curious and less savvy than him criticized his anatomical and physiological point of view, which in their opinion reduced the body's limbs to a machine moved by levers and counter-levers, or the heart to a pump. No doubt, living matter is much more plastic and very complex, but Leonardo's observations represented the first methodical approach to studying nature in general and the human body in particular. Leonardo tried to understand how nature functions and proposed mathematical models that represented the basis of modern physiology and a definitive break with the dogmas of the past. His research on the functions of our body represented the beginning of experimental physiology, a science that received other, fundamental insights, especially concerning blood circulation, by the work of William Harvey, who was a disciple of Fabricius da Acquapendente in Padua.

(see later).

Chapter 2
Bloodletting, an Ancient Therapy

It has taken millennia to understand the composition of blood, and the scarcity of knowledge paralleled the paucity of treatments. One such treatment given long before we understood about blood was Bloodletting (or Phlebotomy*).

Bloodletting was a popular, quite archaic, medical practice that has been used for more than five thousand years. Doctors of the distant past and even those until just over a century ago prescribed bloodletting, often repeatedly given, for almost all conditions, from mental diseases to fevers and various kinds of organic diseases. The purpose, then, was to 'rebalance' the blood humors, which, according to Hippocratic Medicine were phlegm (mucous, sputum), green bile, yellow bile, and blood. With the discovery of blood circulation and respiration, as well as the introduction of blood transfusion (see Chap. 13), bloodletting saw a progressive decline until its virtual cessation at the end of the late nineteenth century. The reasons for the abolition of this long-standing practice are numerous.

Perhaps the most important issue is that its efficacy was never proven. Modern medicine is based on the collection of data and their analysis that led to the development of medical statistics. Using systematic collection of data and methodically observing clinical events before and after treatment, it was documented that bloodletting was not only ineffective for almost all the suggested applications but in most of cases, it was harmful!

During the Middle Ages, bloodletting was performed by priests in monasteries. After a Papal prohibition, it was performed by a new category of workers, the barber-surgeons. These 'sawbones', as they were called, performed all types of surgery, from dental extractions to trauma surgery, but they were also selling miraculous remedies. Doctors themselves had abandoned the practice of bloodletting since many of them were executed or imprisoned by feudal lords when bloodletting didn't have its expected effects. Hence, the barber-surgeons became prosperous in practices other than beard, haircutting, and dental extractions.

G. Mariani et al., *Blood: The Science, History, and Mysteries of Life's Vital Flow*, https://doi.org/10.1007/978-3-031-92481-1_2

In the Eighteenth and Nineteenth centuries, some barber–surgeons specialized in surgical castration before puberty, which led to the persistence of an infantile voice into adulthood. These 'unfortunate' children were called 'castrated' and some of them became real phenomena in the history of music.

Bloodletting, in the absence of effective remedies, was often practiced by the barber-surgeons (Fig. 2.1), and to protect themselves from the risk of imprisonment or execution, they linked the practice to astrology. They claimed that it was better if

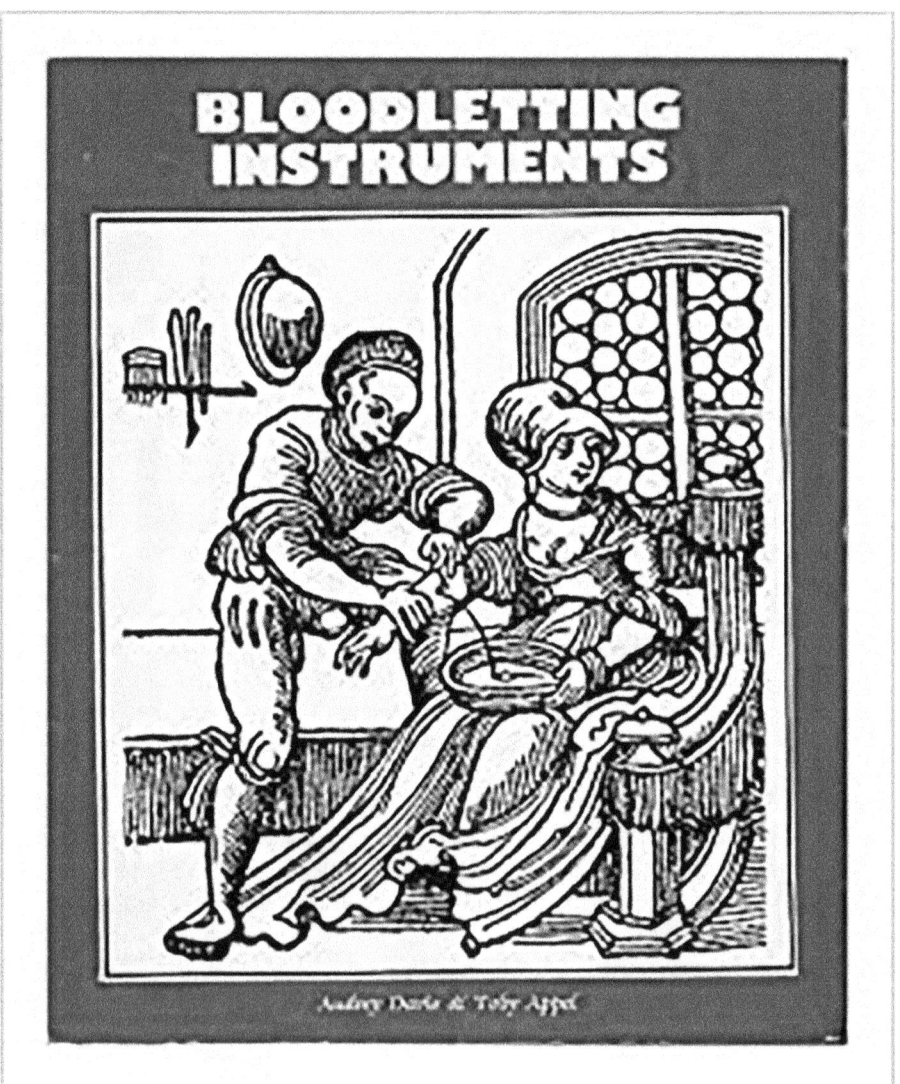

Fig. 2.1 Cover of the book by Audrey Davis, Bloodletting Instruments in the National Museum of History & Technology, 1983 ISBN-10 091549700X

bloodletting was performed, and purgatives* given when astral events were favorable: never when there was a full moon! Bloodletting and purgatives were such universally accepted remedies that the second publication of a medical text was the Bloodletting Calendar of Gutenberg (1462), while the first medical text was the Purgation Calendar (1457). The Bible, the first book ever printed, was published in 1453. The shops of the 'barber-surgeons' were often noticed by passers-by through a small red and white striped column, or a blue, white, and red column displayed outside. The white stripes represented the bandages, the red the arterial blood, and the blue the venous blood. Interestingly, until only a few years ago, this was often seen in the form of rotating illuminated spirals outside barber shops.

To open the veins, bloodletting practitioners used blades that were sharp on both sides. The choice of the vein used depended on the type of illness the 'patient' had. The blood was collected in jars, often made of glass, and the amount was measured. Once the bloodletting was finished, pressure was applied to the wound, and a bandage was placed on it. The amount of blood removed was decided by the operator along with the number of bloodlettings.

In 1645, the rector of the University of Medicine of Paris, Guy Patin, wrote: "There is no remedy in the world that creates so many miracles as bloodletting". Patin was not completely wrong when he said: 'Parisians normally practice few physical exercises, they drink lots of wine and eat a lot and in this way, they become plethoric'. In this condition, 'The most powerful remedy for the plethora* of ensuing illnesses is copious and frequent bloodletting'. Patin identified what we nowadays call the Metabolic Syndrome, with one of its main symptoms being the increased body mass, together with high levels of fats in the blood. Patin was so sure of the efficacy of bloodletting that he repeatedly carried out bloodletting on his wife, his son, and his eighty-year-old brother-in-law. Perhaps Moliere thought of him when he painted a doctor in his comedy 'The Hypochondriac'.

Another bloodletting fanatic was Benjamin Rush, known in Philadelphia as the 'Prince of Bloodletting'. In 1793, during the yellow fever pandemic (an illness caused by a virus), he was so convinced of the efficacy of the practice that he performed bloodlettings and gave purgatives to everyone who entrusted him, seemingly hundreds of people. At the end of the pandemic, he claimed to have saved the town. His excessive pride and vanity were attacked by a journalist who accused him of having fudged his story and hiding the number of deaths as the result of his treatment.

The journalist poked fun at Rush, calling him the Hippocrates of Philadelphia. A long-lasting lawsuit followed and by the end, the journalist was forced to pay 5000 dollars to Rush and was convicted of defamation. However, the journalist continued to advocate that bloodletting had to be abandoned. Shortly after his conviction, a terrible event occurred supporting his beliefs: George Washington became sick with a sore throat, was treated with bloodlettings, and died (1799). In the newspapers, doctors were accused of imprudence and physicians began to realize that bloodletting was not perhaps such an effective treatment. An influential doctor publicly said: 'Old people do not tolerate bloodletting as well as the young ones'.

So even public opinion began to consider that bloodletting was neither effective nor safe. However, despite this the practice continued to be used. Napoleon, who notoriously did not mince his words, after a bloodletting session told a doctor that 'medicine was the science of murders'. Even Mozart died in a state of shock, because of bloodletting and purgatives were given to him for an infective fever. In Italy, there were also bloodletting victims: Camillo Benso, Count of Cavour, the first Italian Premier, had six bloodlettings in four days. It seems that he was treated with bloodletting for tertian malaria with cerebral complications, an absolute contraindication for bloodletting, as in malaria there is no need to remove blood cells since the malaria parasites destroy them! Camillo Benso's death caused a stir even amongst prestigious scientific journals such as The Lancet and The New England Journal of Medicine since it was thought that the cause of his death was bloodletting.

The first circumspect observation that bloodletting was ineffective was made by Pierre-Charles-Alexandre Louis, who can be considered one of the fathers of medical statistics. His work and publications showed that bloodletting was not the panacea for all illnesses. His conclusions were cautious, but the death reported in 1835 were numerous and the data analysis was rigorous.

New generations of medical graduates in the nineteenth century were beginning to be educated using careful symptom analysis, precise medical examination, and new disciplines such as microbiology and the morphological examination of blood and tissues. This led to the progressive abandonment (after 5000 years), of the practice of bloodletting, especially in academic circles and in large cities. The practice persisted in the countryside for a few more decades. Along with standard bloodletting, another practice fell into almost complete disuse: bloodletting with leeches which are big black worms that rely on blood for their nutrients. Leeches were used for the treatment of heart failure until 70–80 years ago.

Box 2.1: Blood and the More Common Diseases According to De Savignac's View in 1861

Blood changes	Related disease
Raised fibrin	Pregnancy, inflammation, rheumatism
Decreased fibrin	Haemorrhage, cachexia, scurvy, purpura
Raised albumin	Phlegmasia, cholera
Decreased albumin	Pregnancy, nephritis, cachexia
Raised red blood cells	Plethora* (excess of blood), feverish states
Decreased red blood cells	Chlorosis (now termed hypochromatic anaemia), anaemias
Raised white blood cells	Liver, spleen and lymph nodes diseases, leukemias
Increase of water	Anaemia and albumin reduction
Reduction of water	Plethora, cholera
Raised salts	Scurvy, haemorrage
Decreased salts	Yellow fever, plague, cholera

Nowadays, the indications for the use of bloodletting are rare, and if really necessary it is performed by specialists using the methods and instruments used for blood donations (i.e. plastic bags, etc.). The only rational indication for bloodletting are Polycythemia Vera, a rare disease where the marrow produces excess red blood cells, and Haemochromatosis, a very rare genetic condition characterized by an excess of iron in the body. In the latter case, removing red blood cells is the simplest way to remove iron. Today, there is also a variant of bloodletting, called 'white bloodletting', which is carried out using diuretics in cases of peripheral edema* or the most severe cases of pulmonary edema.

The basis of modern medicine originated at the end of the nineteenth century when the first classification of illnesses began to appear. The box below shows what it is believed to be one of the first classifications of blood abnormalities, according to the studies of De Savignac, a professor at the University of Toulon, called 'Alterations of the proportions of the basic elements of blood' (Box 2.1).

Chapter 3
Blood, Racism, and Misbeliefs

It seems strange that blood has for so long been used to separate, discriminate, and even cause fights between people.

At the end of the Middle Ages, blood was explicitly thought of as a sign of the purity of a cast. It was when the reigning Spanish family of Castile claimed the superiority of their white race by saying that they had Sangre Azul in their veins, thus implying that they did not mix with the Moors—the Arabs who had settled in Southern Spain. The basis of their claim was that through white skin, veins appeared blue, a color not visible in the Moors who had dark skin. Since then, 'Blue Blood' has been synonymous with Nobility or Royalty. The term became popular in Victorian England and retains the same meaning even today.

The pronouncement of the Castile Family is probably the first example of the many expressions of social and racial differences based on blood, which, needless to say, have no scientific basis! However, there have been numerous pseudoscientists who have worked intensely to document biological differences among races to accumulate proof of the superiority or inferiority of a certain race. Since blood is the most significant and the most accessible among all the tissues, it became the preferred object of investigation. Recently, these works have been collected into a 'school' of thought called Scientific Racism, opinions that have been repeatedly and consistently rebutted. Despite this, the belief still exists that there are genetic and biological differences amongst races that influence (positively or negatively) cognitive skills, intelligence (also the intelligence quotient I.Q.), and courage. This false and pseudoscientific approach is based on the hypothesis, never proven, that races are the result of inherited and unmodifiable genetic traits, neither influenced by environmental factors, nor by genetic mixing.

G. Mariani et al., *Blood: The Science, History, and Mysteries of Life's Vital Flow*, https://doi.org/10.1007/978-3-031-92481-1_3

The 'Aryan' Race

For the Nazis, the concept of the 'purity of blood' and thus 'purity of race', was a poisonous blend of antisemitism and misinterpretation of Darwinism, to prove the existence of the 'Aryan Race', and therefore legitimize the reason to seize and maintain power. To achieve this, they invested in scientific institutions and recruited incompetent individuals to justify their ideologies. One of these individuals was Otto Reche, a Viennese anthropologist, who founded the German Society for the Study of Blood Groups and a journal, 'Population and Race'. Reche, a member of the National-Socialist party, claimed to continue the studies of a great Viennese hematologist who had discovered Blood Groups, 30 years before, Karl Landsteiner (see Chap. 13). Numerous nazi scholars established studies to differentiate between 'Arian' and 'non-Arian' populations (namely Jews and Poles) utilizing blood groups, physical physiognomy, and other characteristics. One of these people even tried to correlate blood groups with the duration of defecation and proposed that blood group A carriers (who wrongly identified with the Aryans) defecated rapidly, while those with blood group B took 40 minutes! In the end, a series of ridiculous studies confirmed (what is now common knowledge) that group A is the most frequent blood group among the English (42%), while group B is more frequent in India (35%). In other populations, there can be a different prevalence of blood groups (see Chap. 13). The results of this anthropological research were never made known: in Berlin, the prevalence of blood groups was similar in both Arians and the Jewish people!

Obviously, during the Nazi era, it was forbidden to transfuse non-Aryan blood into an Aryan: in 1935 a countryside doctor of Jewish belief saved the life of a patient by donating his compatible blood, arm to arm. He was subsequently interned in a concentration camp for six months accused of having 'polluted' the Aryan's blood. Once released, he quickly emigrated.

Reche, on the other hand, continued his studies and teachings in Germany at various universities pushing different ethnic studies. Once the war started, he focussed on ethnic studies of Polish people, who, according to him, were a racial blend, compared to the German, a pure Aryan race. These studies were carried out to demonstrate how much the Aryan race deserved to occupy the Polish land thus justifying the invasion of Poland. At the end of the war, the Nazi anthropologist was arrested by the Americans and served a short detention. In 1959, he was still active as a university lecturer and 'expert anthropologist'. In this capacity, he was involved in the famous trial of Anastasia's recognition as the daughter of Tsar Nicholas II. The lady who initiated the trial said she had escaped death in Ekaterinburg and claimed her rights to the treasure of the Tsars that was in a Swiss bank. By studying the appearance of the woman, Reche expressed his opinion that the woman was undoubtedly Anastasia or, if not, a twin sister. After many years, this legal expertise marked the end of his career: when the bodies of the Romanoffs were found in Ekaterinburg a DNA* investigation clearly showed that the woman was not the daughter of the Tsar; she was not a Romanov, but an impostor!

Blood and Racism Even in Democratic Societies

Blood also caused problems to the champions of democracy. Charles Drew was universally recognized as the founder of the blood donation programs in the USA (Fig. 3.1, this chapter). Drew was an African American from Washington and the eldest of four brothers. His father, a workman, had difficulties in maintaining such a large family, but Charles was able to pursue his studies thanks to his athletic abilities. He won medals as a swimmer and grants as a football player and athlete. However, his dream was to become a doctor. At that time, an African American couldn't have access to an American University, so he enrolled at the University of McGill in Montreal, one of the most prestigious Canadian universities. McGill ranked and still ranks high in Canada amongst all the medical schools. Drew graduated in Medicine as the second in his course and earned a master's degree in Surgery. While still a student and working as a laboratory technician to support himself, he recognized the importance of blood transfusion for surgery and trauma and started studying the separation of plasma and the storage of blood cells. He wrote a voluminous doctoral thesis entitled 'Banking Blood' that sancicipated an innovative concept: 'Blood Banks'. With the outbreak of the Second World War and based on his expertise, he was asked to be head of a program 'Plasma for Britain', which turned out to be a great success. From this, a contentious concern arose: what to do with the blood of Black people? Drew clearly stated that blood was blood and there were no differences related to skin colour. However, the establishment wanted to exclude blood coming from donations of African Americans, and thus, Drew resigned from the Program. A few years into the war the American Red Cross delegated Drew with the task of organizing blood donations for the armed forces. Drew, therefore, organized the donations at the national level. After less than a year, the problem of African-American donations cropped up once again.

Initially, the Red Cross wanted to exclude blood donations from Black people, creating formal racial segregation of donations. Later, following pressures from the armed forces, the Red Cross accepted the donation of 'black blood' but on the condition that it was only given for transfusion to other blacks. This school of thought resulted in a strong backlash in the Northern States. It was, also, the subject of a large report in the New York Times: 'The prejudice against blood from Black individuals is even more difficult to understand if we consider that many white citizens resident in the Southern States were breastfed by black wet nurses. We cannot understand the prejudice that the Red Cross continued to express. Sometimes we wonder if this attitude is compatible with what was going on in the twentieth century which is characterized by strong scientific development'.

It was not only the Red Cross that pursued this discrimination, a serious issue for the image of an organization based on ethical principles, but this issue spread on a national scale. As a result, the blood banks in Baltimore and New Orleans decided to open transfusion centers for only the African American communities, but with very disappointing results. Around that time, an anonymous letter sent to a senator of the Deep South made a sensational splash. The letter expressed the fear that any

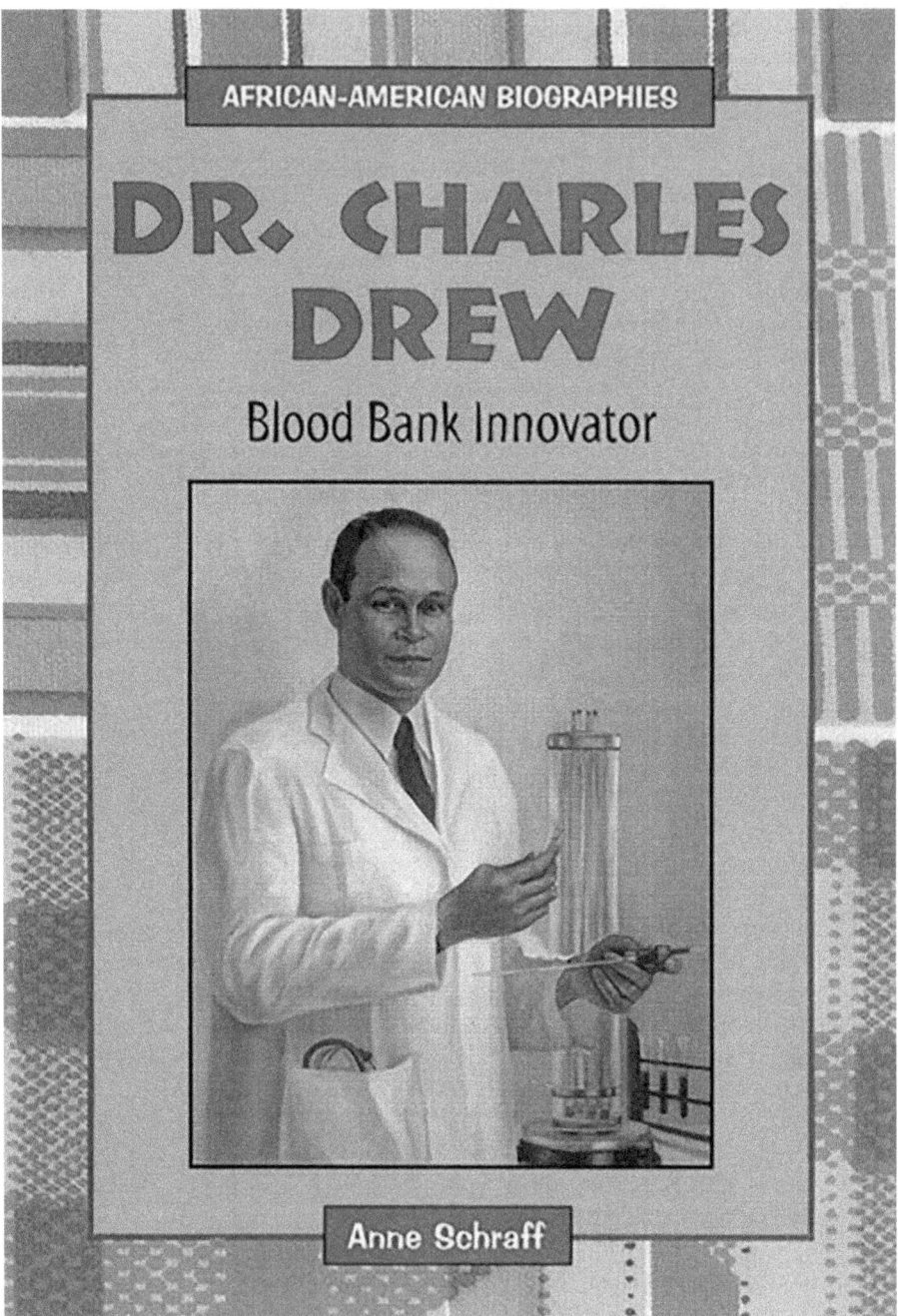

Fig. 3.1 Cover of the book by Anne Schraff celebrating the ingenuity of Charles Drew (Enslow Publishing, LLC, 2003)

blood product coming from races other than white could have deleterious effects on a white recipient. This letter was published in the newspapers and concluded: 'How many whites, if they could have the choice, would prefer to die in a battle rather than receiving plasma from a non-white and so running the risk of becoming the father, the grandfather or the great grandfather of a half-breed, red, black or yellow?' When the Red Cross decided to refuse blood from African Americans in 1941, thousands of letters expressing similar views were sent to members of Congress.

This controversy went viral and three months later it prompted the Red Cross to change its position by accepting blood from African Americans but still maintaining segregation: blood from African Americans had to be transfused to other African Americans. However, more than 120,000 African Americans were fighting in Europe and Asia making the segregation of blood a serious problem from an organizational point of view. In 1943, at the peak of the controversy, a group of university science students published a poster that depicted a soldier being offered two bottles of blood: one from an African American, the other from a white person. The writing said: 'They are the same thing, even science says that. Science has proved through chemical, physical, and microscopic investigations that blood from whites is the same as that from African Americans.' The poster caused a sensation and was published in numerous journals. One of the most appropriate comments made on the stance of the New York students was that the USA, England, and France were fighting a war against Nazi and Fascist countries and therefore a segregational policy by an official institution, the Red Cross, was unacceptable. The American Society of Anthropology wrote an article in the prestigious Journal of the American Medical Association (JAMA) in strong opposition to the discrimination against blood donation between white and black individuals. This concern was shared by the equally prestigious journal 'Science,' in an article entitled 'The segregation of Bloods'. Also, the popular science magazine Scientific American published an article with the title: 'It is not science: the aversion towards non-Caucasian blood is emotional and not based on scientific data'.

This controversy continued through its ups and downs until 1959 when a white patient received blood donated from an African American for open-heart surgery and died from a haemolytic reaction. This unfortunate incident triggered a backlash until it was found that the patient had become immunized against a rare red blood cell antigen* (antigen Kidd) after a previous transfusion from a white donor positive for the Kidd antigen: a clear transfusion error!

Finally, a very strong argument against the discriminatory use of blood transfusions was proposed in an article in the New York Times based on a letter sent by a doctor from the South African Red Cross. The article described how interracial transfusions had been performed in racist South Africa for more than twenty years, without causing any side effects. Blood units donated by white citizens, who represented only 8% of the South African population, would not have been sufficient to cover 95% of the country's needs: the 'black' blood had saved millions of white lives!

In the USA, year after year, de-segregation became the basis of various political administrations, but the process has been very slow. The first move was initiated by Truman when in 1949: the armed forces were de-segregated. However, blood segregation continued until the end of the '70 s in a few Southern States.

Genetics and the Concept of 'Race'

Eight years before Hitler's rise to power, the concept of race and racial separation was disputed by an Editor of the journal 'Scientific American' based on three concepts:

- In the world, a pure race does not exist, the Nordic race is a pure myth.
- Not even the slightest proof exists that one race is potentially more skilled and honest than another one.
- Races blend, a genetic event which is very useful to civilization, i.e. populations gain strength by increasing their gene pool with the mixing of races.

However, the concept of 'race' has caused significant interpretative difficulties amongst geneticists. The 'Homo Sapiens' who emigrated from Africa, mixed with the Neanderthals (200,000–40,000 BC), the Denisovans, and who knows how many other populations of sapiens. This led to a strong expansion of genetic variation. As a result of this re-mixing of Homo Sapiens from various other areas, dark skin became a predominant characteristic feature in Europe and remained such until about 6000 years ago. During the Agricultural Revolution, black skin became prevalent as demonstrated by Cavalli-Sforza, a prominent Italian geneticist. His findings were confirmed by the DNA studies performed on the skeletons of the first homo sapiens (harvester-hunters) found in Spain, Luxembourg, and Hungary, demonstrating that about 8000 years ago, these populations had dark skin. Therefore, at that time, 'Europeans' all had dark skin. Later, different characters (white skin, eye color, etc.) took over first in Scandinavia and then in the rest of Europe. The work of the great historian Frank Snowden demonstrated that in Egypt, ancient Greece, and ancient Rome, ethnic differences were not considered a problem but rather an opportunity for development. Also, slavery paid no attention to skin color. Following these and other studies, most geneticists consider the term 'race' meaningless. Nowadays, in scientific communications, terms like 'ethnic groups' or 'populations' are considered more appropriate. This concept has been reinforced following the completion in 2003 of a massive scientific research program by thousands of scientists all over the world, known as 'The Human Genome Project'. In this global program, the gene that define most human characteristics have all been identified along with the various enzyme molecules that make our bodies function.

However, there are still situations where deeply-rooted discrimination still occurs. In India, even today, the 'Untouchables' (the Dalits) cannot come into contact even with the blood or the cadavers of the 'superior' classes since they would 'contaminate' them. Needless to say, the untouchables cannot donate their blood, a fact that aggravates the serious problem concerning the lack of blood for transfusion in India (the Dalit population comprises about 300 million people). Ethnically speaking, the Dalits are indistinguishable from the 'non-Dalits' or the maharajas: they have the same color of hair, the same physiognomic traits, and obviously, the same blood. This segregation is nowadays against the Indian law, but there remains strong opposition to this important social reform. However, a seed of hope has been planted: in the general elections, India has elected a Dalit as President of the Republic (2017).

It is not well known, but classes of 'Untouchables'are also present in Japan, Burma, Korea, and Tibet with the same problems of segregation.

Chapter 4
Women, Blood, and Prejudices

Blood is the foundation of life, yet women, who are the carriers and guardians of new generations, have a different relationship with blood than men. Their reproductive system is amazing. The villi of the embryo are like roots, eager for oxygen and nutrients captured from the maternal blood and transferred to the fetus through the umbilical cord.

With the maternal blood flowing through the uterus at a rate of roughly 0.6–0.7 liters per minute, the villi in the mature placenta offer an exchange surface area of 10 m². Hence every 6–7 minutes the entire volume of maternal blood passes through the placenta. This relationship between the maternal blood and the blood of the fetus is incredibly complex: none of the maternal blood cells pass through the villi barrier and the system is so well organized that it allows the fetus an autonomous and protected development. Only some antibodies (IgG, Chap. 6) from the maternal blood can pass across the placenta. This provides 'passive' protection after birth against bacteria and viruses, as the antibodies remaining in the circulation of the newborn for only a month or so. We must also consider that in each pregnancy the fetus is like a transplant to the mother because it contains genes derived from the mother but also the father. The fetus could be rejected if the maternal immune cells react with antigens different from her own, i.e. those of the father. However, during pregnancy, a sort of 'immunological tolerance' develops which fortunately prevents a rejection. This occurs mainly, but not exclusively, because the placenta acts as a guardian, stopping the passage of cells in both directions. But, at birth, some blood cells of the offspring can enter the maternal circulation leading to an immune response which cause a problem in future pregnancies.

Despite the vital relationship between women and blood, this has been a source of prejudice and discrimination. The first blood loss during menarche (the first menstrual period), represents one of the most amazing and dramatic transformations from childhood to womanhood but has suffering in young women. Stories collected by a Naturalist in the 1800s report that the Innuit people locked up girls in an igloo

© The Author(s), under exclusive license to Springer Nature Switzerland AG 2025
G. Mariani et al., *Blood: The Science, History, and Mysteries of Life's Vital Flow*, https://doi.org/10.1007/978-3-031-92481-1_4

during their menarche until they reached 'normality'. Native American tribes were more civil: during the menarche, girls stayed in a tent with their eldest sisters, mothers, and grandmothers, and this was a custom during the menstruation periods.

Considering menstruation, in the Bible, the term 'impurity' is used, and it is emphasized that women should not touch anything during their periods. Aristotle indicated that menstruation was evidence of a woman's inferiority, and considered the phenomenon 'supernatural', because it was incomprehensible. Plinius the Old thought that everything a woman touched during their period 'went off': i.e. wine became vinegar and iron became rusty.

Even today, television commercials for painkillers make use of the idea that women are disagreeable and irritable during their periods. And in the English language, there is an old term used to mean menstruation, 'the curse'.

An English journalist, very active in battles for women's rights who probably suffered a lot during her periods, wrote: "What kind of role in evolution can pain have that affects 50% of the population who lose blood 12 times per year?" While another journalist considers that menstruation is not a problem: "Menstruation is not my problem, but the problem for others. If somebody (a man) does not tolerate menstruation, he does not tolerate women".

Simply put, menstrual blood is the manifestation of regulated bleeding that contains cellular remnants of the uterine wall following a process of tissue renewal. It is a way, the getting rid of tissue each month prepares the uterus to accept a fertilized egg!!

In a recent publication (see references), we presented the results of a study on the quantity of blood lost by women during their periods. The result, obtained from a large cohort of women, was transformed into the first patented method for assessing the amount of iron lost during menstruation. It was concluded that if the loss of iron is more than 2.5 milligrams per period, anemia is inevitable, it is only a matter of time. In fact, in the case of heavy periods, more than 10 milligrams of iron can be lost, and so all the iron stored in the body would be lost in less than two years. Anemia (see Chap. 10), according to the WHO, is one of the most important priorities for public health: it affects 1 billion and 621 million individuals worldwide. In 800 million of these (approx. 50%), anemia is caused by iron deficiency and females account for about 80%. Severe anemia causes not only paleness and profound fatigue, but also hair loss, nail frailty, dry skin, and discomfort of the mouth mucosa*. It should be taken into account in most of the cases anemia is avoidable with a precocious diagnosis and a simple treatment!

In previous centuries, a common and very severe problem of public health was represented by postpartum hemorrhages (events that can occur from one [early] to twelve [late] days after delivery). This had been a very serious issue because it was associated with a very high mortality rate, close to 100%. Most of the early transfusion attempts were put in place to save these unfortunate mothers. In recent years, mortality is still high in developing countries: almost 300,000 deaths every year compared to 2200 in industrialized countries.

Fibroids can also cause uterine hemorrhages or heavy menstruation (metrorrhagia* or menorrhagia* respectively) which are often causes of anemia and unnecessary hysterectomies (surgical removal of the uterus). It was reported that in the USA, 2/3 of the interventions of hysterectomies are unnecessary, considering that bleeding can be kept under control with pharmacological treatments or with minimally invasive surgery.

Another problem, particularly relevant to women, concerns the venous circulation in the lower extremities. There are no differences in the venous system between the sexes, but pregnancies and poorly exercised leg muscles make the veins in females more vulnerable. In more detail, vein valves often become ineffective if the abdominal venous pressure is excessive, as in obesity or during pregnancy. Impaired blood flow in the veins results in the appearance of varicose veins (the bulging of superficial veins remaining filled with blood). There are two types of varicose veins, the deep and the superficial ones: the deep represent a serious problem whilst the superficial ones represent mostly an aesthetic problem.

Venous thrombosis was once thought to be an inflammatory phenomenon and therefore was called phlebitis. The most important issue is the fact that when and where an impaired venous circulation develops the occurrence of thromboembolism is likely to occur. These problems can be prevented with the adoption of a healthy lifestyle aimed at protecting the veins and maintaining appropriate body weight. This implies regular physical activity, keeping body weight compatible with one's height and age, and avoiding smoking. The presence of a toned and active musculature around the veins considerably helps the venous blood return.

Part II
Understanding Blood: The Science

Chapter 5
The Discovery of Blood

It all started with the development of the microscope that allowed the observer to see really small objects. The development of lenses with their magnifying properties was essential for this. Although lenses had been around for thousands of years (Seneca tells of Emperor Nero using a lens-shaped emerald to see better the performance of the gladiators) the invention of glasses (spectacles) as a practical daily appliance goes back to the Florentine Salvino degli Armati, who in the thirteenth century made glass prototypes, but kept his invention secret for a long time as a family legacy. In the sixteenth century Zacharias Jansen, found that he could see tiny things not otherwise visible by stacking the lenses in a tube: he was given credit for the invention of the microscope. However, Robert Hook, in the mid-seventeenth century, made the most of this invention and wrote a book (Micrographia), showing sketches he had drawn of the shapes of snow crystals, hairs of flies, wings of butterflies, and the structure of cork. He had noticed that cork was made up of structures like wood sacs containing air, (this is why cork floats) for which he proposed the term '**cell**', a term borrowed from the name given to the small monastic rooms. At that time, microscopes could only magnify 30 times (scientifically: powers 30×).

Antoni von Leeuwenhoek, a Dutch cloth trader was eager to analyze the structure and weave of his cloth. He created a new microscope with a higher magnification power of up to 200 (200x). With this improved device, he started to observe the invisible world. Antoni enjoyed taking part in medical meetings that were held in Delft, in the Netherlands; there, he met a doctor member of the Royal Society of London, who was amazed by Antoni's scientific findings. Once back in London, the doctor discussed Antoni's observations with the members of the Royal Society, and in 1668, Von Leeuwenhoek also was nominated a Member of the Society. So, this Dutch cloth trader put together his observations and sent them to London with the result that many of these were published in the 'records' of that renowned Scientific body. In Europe, he became so popular that even some royals visited him to have a look at his invisible world. Among them, Frederick I of Prussia, Queen Mary of England, and the Tsar Peter the Great visited his shop where he performed

G. Mariani et al., *Blood: The Science, History, and Mysteries of Life's Vital Flow*, https://doi.org/10.1007/978-3-031-92481-1_5

his experiments. Von Leeuwenhoek had shown the Tsar the capillaries in a fishtail. Peter the Great was so enthusiastic about the visit, which lasted some hours, that he warmly congratulated him: the visit ended with an exchange of gifts and Von Leeuwenhoek donated a microscope to the Tsar.

Among the observations Antoni submitted to the Royal Society in London was the first description of the red blood cells. He described this finding: 'Taking a little bit of blood from my hand, I observed that it consists of small globules'. He said that these were 'round-shaped' and moved through the 'crystalline humidity of water': in addition to the globules, he had discovered plasma, the fluid through which globules flow. He was also able to measure the size of the globules calculating that they were 25,000 times smaller than a grain of sand. A great researcher indeed! He had invented a way to measure the infinitely small, using the grain of sand as a 'standard'. Antoni also described the colorless globules and realized that blood, after a few minutes outside the body, changed its status, becoming semi-solid, that is, formed a clot. In total, von Leeuwenhoek sent 400 letters to London and produced around 100 microscopes which he jealously guarded. What is vitally important, is that his drawings and observations sent to the Royal Society, can still be read. He was the forerunner of 'the scientific publications'. It was not until 200 years later (1840–70), that hemoglobin, giving blood its red color, was discovered.

Paul Ehrlich took the observations of van Leeuwenhoek further into the science of blood by using cloth dyes to visualize the colorless 'white' globules (which we now call white blood cells). He gave names to the members of the white cell family, taking into account the acquired color when bathed in certain dyes. Using the Greek word 'phil' which means love, affinity in this case, he distinguished eosinophils, cells liking an acid dye of color red (eosin), from basophils, those liking a basic-dark dye color, and finally, from neutrophils—those liking a neutral color (grey).

The term 'tissue' was used to indicate a group of cells with similar functions (muscular tissue, nervous tissue, connective tissue). The staining methods of Ehrlich triggered a revolution in medicine. Since then, different dyes have been used to examine biological samples. This led to the identification of different cells, tissues, and their functions in the body: in this way, the science that studies tissues under the microscope, Histology, was born and derived its name from the Greek "istòs", which means canvas.

So, by using the given dyes at standard concentrations, it became possible to differentiate normal tissues from those that were abnormal (pathological) and to study samples in a standard way, whether in Frankfurt, London, Paris, or Rome. Thus, by using the same scientific language, the same instruments (microscopes), and the same reagents (dyes), doctors could finally compare their results!

Following Antoni and Paul Ehrlich's initial studies, it became possible to compare scientific observations in different countries and places within the same country: international scientific literature was born. Paul Ehrlich also invented chemotherapy* and diseases could finally have a 'specific' treatment. It was the beginning of the twentieth century and the beginning of the modern medicine, based on standard diagnostic procedures (with dyes) and treatments (with chemotherapies and immunotherapies).

Table 5.1 Summary of the discoveries that led to our understanding of blood

Author	Discoveries	Time
Zacharias Jansen	A microscope by stacking lenses in a tube	End of the sixteenth century
Robert Hook	Improved the microscope (20×—30×) and published the first observations of the invisible	Mid seventeenth century
Antoni Von Leeuwenhoek	Created several functional microscopes (200 x) and started to share his observations with a Medical Society	Circa 1660
Paul Ehrlich	Introduced the use of dyes to distinguish between different cells and their organelles	Circa 1870

It was thanks to Ehrlich's observations of the shape, color, and types of granules in blood cells that the science of blood—Hematology, was born, an independent science both from the experimental and clinical point of view (Table 5.1). In addition, Hematology is one of the few disciplines requiring combined clinical and laboratory expertise.

Paul Ehrlich also made fundamental discoveries in immunology (see Chap. 7).

Chapter 6
The Composition of Blood, Cells and Plasma

Our blood is made of cells suspended in a liquid called plasma. We will first talk about the red blood cells and subsequently of the different types of white cells that can be identified by the dyes of Paul Ehrlich. Cells of the blood are also different in shapes and sizes (volumes), data that are very useful to identify them.

We carry out laboratory blood tests to help in the diagnosis of what is wrong with us. To examine the blood cells the tube required to collect blood withdrawn from our veins (peripheral blood) needs to contain an 'anticoagulant' to stop it from clotting. This then allows the cells to be analyzed in a 'particle counter' that measures their volume and the type of light they scatter in a beam projected at them based on treatment with cellular stains (Ehrlich stains!). Hemoglobin (Hb or Hgb) carried by the red blood cells is measured by a chemical method and represents by far the most accurate, precise, and reproducible measurement (in gram/dL [deciliter]). It is also one of the most important parameters to measure: we breathe through our hemoglobin!

The electrical impulses generated by the particle counters are analyzed by a computer and the data is displayed in the form of graphs. Other parameters can be measured that are useful to help the doctors in making a diagnosis. The most important is the hematocrit (Ht or Hct), which results from the sum of the volumes of all the blood cells. It is expressed in percent of the total blood volume (normally 45%) and is composed mainly of red cells (99%). The remaining volume (55%) represents the liquid part of the blood, the 'plasma' (see later).

The Cells Now, let's concentrate on the cells in the blood (Fig. 6.1).

G. Mariani et al., *Blood: The Science, History, and Mysteries of Life's Vital Flow*, https://doi.org/10.1007/978-3-031-92481-1_6

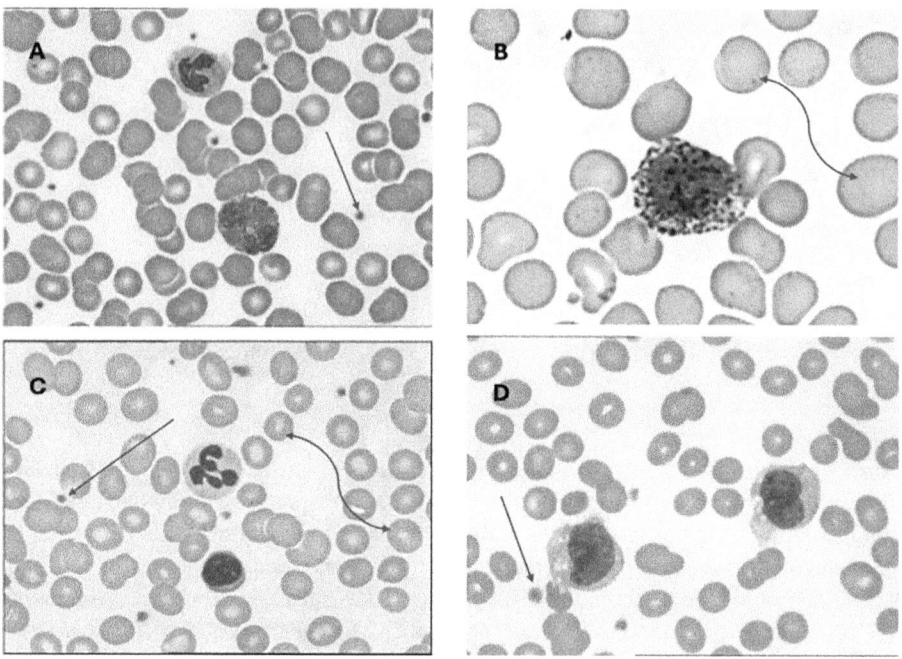

Fig. 6.1 Blood cells. Three main populations are distinguished: white blood cells (WBC), red blood cells (RBC), and platelets. (**a**) Neutrophil (top) and eosinophil (bottom), (**b**) basophil, (**c**) neutrophil (top) and lymphocyte (bottom), (**d**) monocytes. Platelets are shown with straight arrows and red blood cells with curved arrows

RBC

RBC is the acronym used to indicate one of the 25 billion red elements circulating in our vessels. An alternative term of the RBC is Erythrocyte*. This element (is not a real cell since it has no nucleus*), has a strange shape, that of a biconcave disk. Its diameter is 7.5–8.7 microns or μm (micro-meter), and its thickness varies from 1.7 to 2.2 μm. The RBC shape presents the largest possible surface to facilitate oxygen exchange between hemoglobin and the tissues. And each RBC is the proud carrier of as many as 280×10^6 molecules of hemoglobin (280 million molecules, yes, you have read this correctly!), all wrapped efficiently within its membrane. The membrane is made up of proteins containing sugar chains that are determinants for the blood groups (see Chap. 13). One of the most important characteristics of an RBC is its elasticity, which enables it to fold and squeeze through the small capillaries and to return to its standard shape in the veins. And it takes only 30 seconds, on average, to do the grand tour, from the heart and back to it. Thirty seconds is sufficient for a body at rest, but if we are running, then its speed increases up to five times since the need for oxygen and nutrients increases. However, not all the RBCs follow the same path: some enter the coronary vessels to feed the heart, others stop halfway at the kidneys, and still others reach the tip of the foot, and from there, laboriously, come back up following a pathway of about 2 m (Chap. 9). Sometimes, RBCs may see a little bit of sun when they pass under the skin (hemoglobin contributing to the skin's rosy appearance). Other times, they flow in total darkness, and in the case of brain circulation, they can even perceive the high-frequency buzz of neurons and synapses. Their job is rather monotonous, always the same: downloading oxygen and uploading carbon dioxide, but their speed can significantly change in the different parts of the circulation. RBCs are initially pushed (in the arteries) by a high pressure, which is measured in millimeters of mercury (mmHg), whereas in the veins, the pressure is much lower, measured in centimeters of water (Chap. 9). During the passage through the capillaries, the hemoglobin releases oxygen (O_2) into the tissues and captures carbon dioxide (CO_2) that is carried to the lungs and released into the atmosphere.

The muscles, which require a large amount of oxygen to carry out their work, have an additional 'specialized' system: they use a protein similar to hemoglobin, called myoglobin, which transfers oxygen to the mitochondria (from Greek mitos = wire and chondrion = granule for their shapes), the energy powerhouse of the cells. In these amazing organelles, there are other containing iron oxygen carriers, the cytochromes. Incidentally, the number of mitochondria varies depending on the type of cell, for example, there are none in the red blood cells, few in some cells of the immune system but up to 2000 in liver cells. Unlike the red cells of amphibians, fishes, reptiles, and birds which have a small nucleus, the RBCs of mammals don't have a nucleus.

Red blood cells circulate in the bloodstream many times, for an average of 120 days; if you make the calculation, 120 (days) $\times$ 24 (hours) $\times$ 60 (minutes) $\times$ 60 (seconds) $\times$ 30 (seconds), it is more than one billion times! When their energy reserves are finally depleted, they are trapped and destroyed in the spleen and their constituents are recycled (iron above all). This is a very effective process as the spleen's macrophages* destroy about five million RBC per second which will then be replaced by approximately the same number of young fit fellows called Reticulocytes—Ret. These are the RBCs that have just been produced by the marrow (see Chap. 8).

WBC (White Blood Cells)

The Granulocytes

This family of circulating cells was initially called microphages* as opposed to macrophages (see later), then granulocytes since they have granules in their cytoplasm*. These were the first cells identified by Paul Ehrlich; they have a diameter of 12–14 μm and are the most prevalent white cells in the blood.

Paul Ehrlich's observations on granulocytes, although not known at the time, turned out not only to be the birth of hematology, but also the birth of immunology, for which he and the Russian scientist Ilya Metchnikoff (who discovered the macrophage) received the Nobel Prize in 1908.

We now identify the neutrophil as having small pale granules, the eosinophil having numerous prominent orange microspheres, and the basophil being covered by dark blue spheres (see Fig. 6.1). These cells have a relatively short life span of only a few hours when in the blood and a few days when in the tissues. Their number in the blood varies, being roughly 2000, 200 or 20 per microliter (µL) of blood, respectively. Once produced and circulating in the blood stream, these cells do not show any cell division. The neutrophil is clearly a very important player in immunity, and one way it does this is through release of the contents of its segmented nucleus by spreading webs (called NETs), like those of the gladiators. These webs are composed of DNA, enzymes, and sticky proteins that, by surrounding bacteria and fungi, prepare them for the hungry Macrophages (from Greek phagein—to eat). The red-headed eosinophil rushes to the sites where there is an attack by parasites or inflammation of an allergic nature. This cell contains many cytokines* (chemical protein mediators) that transmit messages to other cells during the course of immune reactions. The basophil is also involved in inflammation but releases anticoagulant and vasodilative substances. All members of the Phil family play a role in immunity with the neutrophils, in particular, being in the front line of defense are good at 'eating' bacteria, viruses, fungi and killing them.

Monocytes and Macrophages

The other front-line defenders are the large and aggressive cells belonging to the Macrophage family. In the blood, these cells are seen as 'Monocytes' (Monos) with a diameter of 15–20 µm. Macrophages go around grabbing and eating anything they deem foreign or strange. There are fewer monocytes than the neutrophils in the blood, but the bone marrow continuously renews them and most of them migrate to and settle in the tissues.

When in the tissues, these cells become tissue macrophages, which mainly reside in the spleen, lymph nodes, liver, nervous tissue, and skin but are also found in other tissues and are involved in homeostasis. When they enter the various tissues of the body, the monocytes become specialized depending on the tissue environment. In essence, their job in all tissues is to attack and 'eat' bacteria, viruses, dead cells, and tumor cells. They also have a strong metabolic activity as witnessed by the high number of mitochondria that they possess. During inflammation, macrophages besiege the area to try to contain it. But macrophages have other sophisticated functions as that of sending information to the lymphocytes about what they contain after doing their job. This starts a 'specific' immune response, such as the production of antibodies. Circulating Monos have a short life—just 1 or 2 days, whilst the majority migrate into tissues to become macrophages and there have a longer life—from 1 month to a year.

Lymphocytes

Finally, there is the mysterious world of the small Lymphs (Lymphocytes): although they all look the same under the microscope, they have several different functions. Some of them can sense everything around them, some are killer cells able to attack foreign invaders and some act as antibody* factories. Some also have a strong memory of an invaders that has previously entered the body. This mysterious army with amazing skills can circulate in the blood without ever getting tired and can also live in the various organs of the immune system—the spleen and lymph nodes and also in other places in the body including the intestine, genitourinary tract, and lungs which are all the main sites of entry of infectious microbes. Some have a very long life but because they all look the same it is very difficult to determine their age.

Moreover, their nucleus contains a large amount of DNA, containing a huge amount of information. Although being such an important population of cells, there are relatively few in circulation (only around 30% of the total white blood cells). However, nothing could be more misleading since there are between 10 and 1000 billion in the entire body, and if put together, will make up about the size of a soccer ball. In the marrow, there are few lymphocytes making up only about 15% of all the marrow cells. This number includes 'tribes' of different cell populations that have different jobs to do. But, how can we identify these different tribes of lymphocytes if they all look the same under the microscope?

As we have discussed, they have various and complex functions in both innate* and acquired immunity*. Each member of a tribe (or population), has multiple antennae and sensors on their (outer cell) surface (Fig. 6.1) with which they receive and send information. They are like the eyes and ears of the cell. Today, we identify lymphocytes by using artificially made antibodies that precisely recognize these particular and very important sensors that are called "Receptors*". These artificial antibodies, combined chemically with fluorescent substances of different colors, allow cells to be identified using devices called Particle Counters (similar to those counting blood cells). By doing this, we can recognize the various tribe members and their function(s). This procedure, called flow cytometry*, is both qualitative and quantitative and is of paramount importance for diagnosing blood diseases. In fact, by using different antibodies in combination, it is possible to identify 'malignant' cells that mimic the ontogeny stages of blood cells. Using a metaphor; the different tribe members have a *number plate*, like cars. These identifiers allow one to distinguish the tribe precursors from one another and to identify diverse tumors. The number plates are called 'Cluster Determinants' (CD*), or CD markers (Table 6.1). To date, 400 CD markers (number plates) have been identified using specific antibodies, with more and more being defined. However, cells have more than one CD marker, and therefore their identification is best based on a combination of more than one CD marker.

Cells are told what to do through biological messengers called, cytokines. Messages are transmitted inside the cell from membrane cytokine receptors. Inside the cell, metabolic pathways are triggered, leading to cell activation and the production of proteins/enzymes or even cell death.

Table 6.1 Cluster determinants (CD) of some cells

Cell	CD
T lymphocytes	CD1
Thymocytes	CD2
T lymphocytes	CD3
T helper lymphocytes	CD4
T cytotoxic or suppressor lymphocytes	CD8
B lymphocyte precursors	CD10
B lymphocytes	CD19
B cell lymphomas	CD20
Monocytes	CD33
Endothelial cells and platelets	CD31
Acute myeloid leukemia	CD33
Hematopoietic stem cells* after birth	CD34
Platelets	CD41 and CD42
Natural killer lymphocytes	CD16 (CD56)
Monocytes and macrophages	CD115
Pluripotent precursors of hematopoiesis	CD123
Endothelial cells	CD141
Tissue factor (initiator of coagulation)	CD142
Rh antigen (D)	CD240
Multiple myeloma, plasma cell tumor	CD269

Receptors on the cell surface may also act as 'ligands' that allow them to bind other cells, antibodies, hormones or proteins that signal biological events. Some ligands display adhesive properties that are important for joining cells to one another.

A very small tribe of lymphs can be distinguished from other lymphs in the blood since they are a little bit larger (10–15 μm vs. 6–9 μm), have chains of red granules, and have functions like those of the other cells of innate immunity. These types of Lymphs are called 'Natural Killers' (NK). These cells directly attack foreign cells, especially tumor cells and cells that are infected with viruses. Their number plate is CD16 (see Table 6.1).

Now, let's talk about the main tribes of lymph, the T and B lymphocytes. B lymphs were first identified in birds by the anatomist Girolamo Fabricio d'Aquapendente [1537–1619] in the now-called 'Bursa of Fabricius', hence the lettering 'B'. Later, B lymphs in mammals were conveniently found to originate in the Bone Marrow. Their number plate contains both CD19 and CD20 and their main function is the production of antibodies. T lymphs also originate from the marrow but are re-programmed in the Thymus (hence the lettering 'T') to learn the coordination of adaptive immunity. T cells are also very active in protecting us from viruses. Another very important function is that of discriminating between the organism's cells ('self') and cells from different organisms e.g. microbes or transplanted cells from someone else ('non-self'). We don't want these T cells to go around killing our own 'self'-cells!!

A very significant part of the mammalian DNA (also found in Neanderthal man who lived between 400,000 and 40,000 years ago), contains many genes with multiple forms (alleles) grouped together on chromosome 6, which forms the Major Histocompatibility Complex (MHC). This gene complex is fundamental for the functioning of our immune system. The proteins expressed by the genes of the MHC locus allow the identification of 'non-self' molecules as one of its main roles.

Furthermore, T lymphocytes (all bearing the CD3 number plate) are divided into two large families, both originating in the thymus: the helper CD4 and the cytotoxic CD8 cells.

As outlined before, Lymphocytes may have more than one CD number. Some of them are shown in Table 6.1. The CD numbers of cell populations other than lymph are also shown in this table.

The morphological aspects and the cluster determinant of a cell or a given cell clone is denominated Immunophenotype.*

Important to note that white Blood Cells & Platelets make up only 5% of the whole blood volume (Fig. 6.2).

How do the different cells fit into the overall immune system?

The granulocytes, monocytes, and macrophages are some of the many types of cells of the innate or 'natural immune system', the first to respond to microbes that enter the body. On the other hand, the different tribes (types) of lymphocytes are part of the adaptive immune system, which is where most of the memory against microbes is stored but takes longer to get into action.

That is, after the infection* with a particular microbe, if an individual becomes infected against the same microbe at a later date there will be a faster and more efficient immune response against it (i.e. the immune system remembers the specific infective agent). Whereas most cells of the innate immune system are found in the bloodstream, lymphocytes and their tribes are mainly concentrated within specific lymphoid organs and tissues. However, they do recirculate from the blood to the lymph and in the lymphoid organs and then back into the bloodstream (Chap. 9).

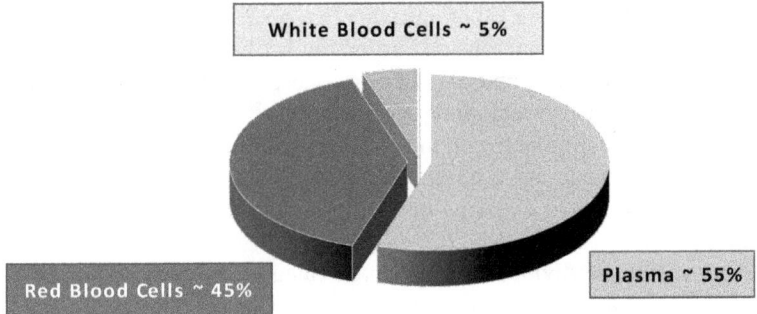

Fig. 6.2 Proportions of blood constituents

Platelets

These are small discs that, in normal conditions, circulate in the blood (Fig. 6.2). However, if provoked, protrusions on their surface will rise (like those of an urchin in danger) and cause them to stick to one another. Platelets are tiny, 3–4 microns (μm), and about 20 times fewer than the RBCs: there are about 150,000–350,000 of them/μL of blood. Platelets have no nucleus, but, unlike RBCs, have a short life, of only 2–3 weeks, after which they are captured by the macrophages in the spleen. When a vessel wall is damaged or ruptured, platelets call and recruit other platelets. From biconvex-shaped discs (like those of a disc thrower) they change their shape into small spheres, send out protrusions, shoot out enzymes, and attract plasma proteins. These complex mechanisms induce the formation of a compact network. On the surface of this network, clotting proteins become involved which strengthens the plug and this tight net stops the blood from oozing out of the vessel. Finally, platelets involve neutrophils in their activity.

PLASMA: The Liquid Fraction of Blood

So far, we have described the cells of the blood, which roughly represent 45% of its volume (Fig. 6.2). The remaining 55% consists of a liquid part called Plasma (which has nothing to do with the fourth state of matter, the term used by physicists to define an ionized gas).

Plasma is a yellowish fluid where the blood cells swim. It contributes up to 25% (3 L in a 70 kg individual) of extracellular fluids while 73% (14 L in a 70 kg individual) is made up of the interstitial fluids located outside blood vessels and the final 2% is made up of the lymph, the fluid drained from the various organs and tissues (Fig. 6.3).

Plasma is in equilibrium with the interstitial fluids since the salts and most proteins can pass via an active transfer mechanism through the capillary walls. Plasma is made up of around 92% water, the remainder being a combination of proteins (around 7%), inorganic salts (sodium, potassium, chloride, calcium, phosphorus), lipids (fats) of different types, other nutrients (amino acids), and, finally, from waste products such as the chylomicrons and other yields of cell metabolism.

Plasma also carries trace amounts of hormones, enzymes, and other substances that are required to service remote organs. Overall, it can be regarded as a communication system, operating between the cells and tissues of the body.

Therefore, we can retrieve a great deal of useful information from just carrying out a blood test. Serum is a plasma-derived product that spontaneously undergoes the clotting process.

Plasma proteins are divided into two main categories: Albumins and Globulins. These are defined based on serum electrophoresis (Fig. 6.4).

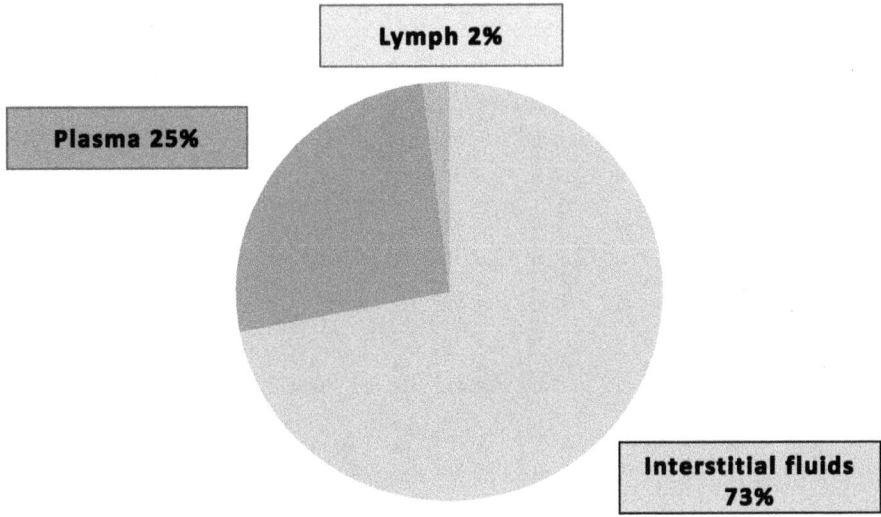

Fig. 6.3 Proportions of extracellular fluids

Albumins represent a very homogeneous class of proteins comprising 55% or circa 3.5–4.5 g/deciliter (dL). By contrast, globulins (2.5–3.0 g/dL) are heterogeneous and include proteins such as antibodies (circulating immunoglobulins IgG, IgA, IgM, and IgE), coagulation factors, lipoproteins, haptoglobin, transferrin, C-Reactive Protein (CRP) and other components with different functions. The globulins are distinguished by the Greek alphabet letters: alpha, beta, and gamma depending on their position after applying an electrical charge to them (electrophoresis—Fig. 6.4). Apart from the antibodies, the liver produces most of the plasma proteins. Many of the plasma proteins are described in Table 6.2.

Albumin is one of the main proteins produced by the liver; around 12 g daily (about 1/3rd of the albumen contained in a hen's egg). The amount of albumin in the plasma is a very important factor since this quiet and hard-working protein contributes to many regulatory mechanisms of our body.

Acute phase proteins (or acute phase reactants) are a group of proteins with different functions, their concentration in the blood increases in response to inflammation, tissue damage, and tumors. There are many of them, but the most well-known are C-reactive protein (CRP), fibrinogen, Von Willebrand factor (vWF), and haptoglobin. The primary function of CRP (which is produced by the liver) is to aid in the phagocytosis of bacteria and is commonly used as an alarm bell in response to inflammation and tumors.

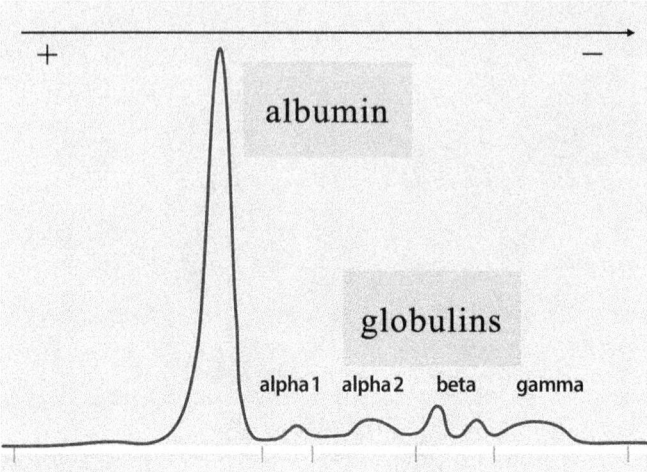

Fig. 6.4 Serum electrophoresis: when a drop of serum is submitted to an electric charge on a 'strip' of special paper (top right of the figure), its proteins are separated into Albumin (the high peak) and Globulins comprising all the other smaller 'humps' called α1 and 2, β1 and 2 and γ. These humps contain all the other proteins or lipoproteins present in the serum

Antibodies

Antibodies belong to a category of globulins (mostly within the gamma fraction) and represent one of the most powerful weapons of Acquired Immunity* or Humoral Immunity*. They are also called Immuno-globulins (Ig). Studies on antibodies began in 1890 when Kitasato Shibasaburö described a blood entity directed to tetanus and diphtheria toxins. A year later, Ehrlich coined the term antikörper to identify those plasma components that were able to bind pathogens. But it was only in the 1920s that Michael Heidelberg and Oswald Avery discovered that antibodies had a protein nature. Anything that is attacked by or binds to antibodies is referred to by the generic name of antigen (bacteria, viruses, foreign substances, or allergens).

When the immune system goes wrong, antibodies can even attach to our own 'self' cellular components. This can cause serious illnesses (autoimmune diseases).

Antibodies are produced by B lymphocytes and Plasma cells; plasma cells derive from B lymphocytes and are specialized for the specific function of producing, only one antibody type in each cell. Moreover, antibodies communicate with the cells of the Immune and the Complement Systems through the tail of their Y-like structure (Fig. 6.5). Antibodies are found in the plasma of circulating blood, on mucosal surfaces such as in the mouth and other parts of the gastrointestinal system, and on the surface of B lymphocytes. Here they act as receptors that attach to foreign 'antigens' and stimulate the B lymphocytes to become plasma cells. Many soluble antibodies are also able to stick to a variety of other cells which are responsible for important reactions in the immune system. A typical B lymphocyte has from 50,000 to 100,000 membrane antibodies on its surface.

Table 6.2 Main proteins found in the plasma and their functions

Protein	What it does
Insulin	Regulates sugar utilisation
GM-CSF	Stimulates production of granulocytes and monocytes
G-CSF	Stimulates granulocyte production
Myoglobin	Acts as the respiratory pigment in muscle
Erythropoietin (EPO)	Stimulates red cell production
Tissue factor (TF)	Initiates coagulation
Factors VII, IX, X	Enzymes involved in coagulation
Haemoglobin	Carries oxygen in red blood cells
Albumin	Retains water in the blood and carries hormones and drugs
Factor II	Involved in blood coagulation
Plasmin	The enzyme that dissolves the clot
IgG	Four sub-classes*: IgG1, IgG2, IgG3, IgG4; involved in immune protection; mainly in tissues
IgA	Involved in immune protection; antibody secreted mainly at mucosal surfaces*
IgE	Involved in immune protection; protection at mucosal surfaces, important in acute inflammation but also main antibody causing allergies*
IgM	Involved in immune protection; the largest of the antibodies and made first in an antibody response*
Haptoglobin	Binds free hemoglobin in the plasma
Fibrinogen	Raw material to build a clot
VonWillebrand factor	Facilitates platelet adhesion, aggregation, and stabilizing factor for factor VIII, multifunctional hemostasis protein

There are five types (classes) of antibodies, identified with the prefix Ig (Immunoglobulin): IgG, IgA, IgM, IgE, and IgD (Fig. 6.5; IgE and IgD are not shown, their structure is similar), made up of two light and two heavy chains. IgM antibodies are the first to be made against pathogens which is called the primary immune response, followed by the IgGs, produced in larger and larger amounts (called the secondary or memory response). It is this memory response that explains how vaccination works, a discovery made by Edward Jenner in the late eighteenth century. Vaccination has saved many, many lives and has been carried out since its discovery.

Acquired immunity has a rapid phase (IgM mediated) followed by a robust IgG-mediated phase, both being highly specific. IgD together with IgM on the surface of the B lymphs act as the sensors that recognize foreign antigens that leads to the secretion of different antibody types by B lymphs.

There is a kind of division of labor between the different secreted antibody types. IgM antibodies work inside the circulatory system whilst IgG antibodies present in the blood can easily leave the circulation and are efficient at attacking pathogens in the tissues. On the other hand, IgA antibodies prevent the attack at the mucosal surfaces, the main entrances of microbes into the body (respiratory, intestinal, and urogenital), and neutralize the pathogens; the same happens with the IgE, which is

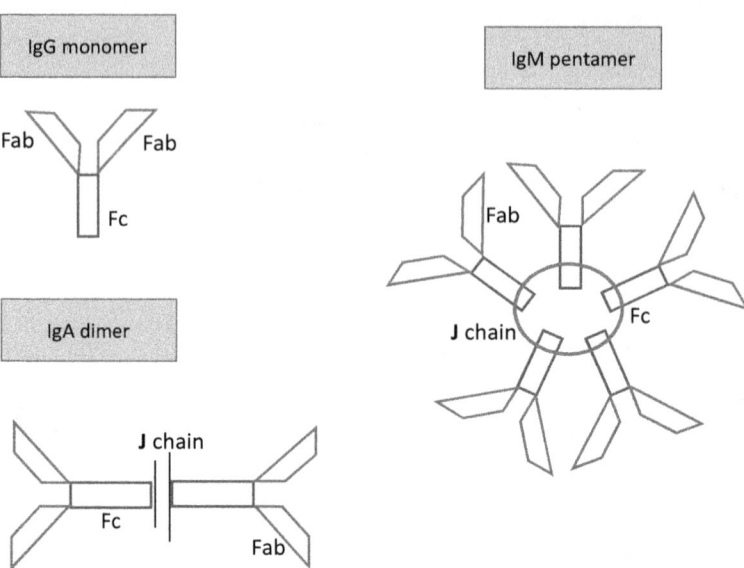

Fig. 6.5 The immunoglobulins: an antibody molecule is made up of two parts. The specificity is present in the Fab (Red in the diagram) and the biological activity i.e. binding to cells and activating complement is located in the Y tail, the Fc part (Blue in the diagram). The J chain (joining chain) attaches the antibodies in dimers (IgA) and pentamers (secreted IgM)

important in attacking worms found in the intestine and in sustaining other allergic reactions.

There are differences among the antibodies which are related to the way they attack the pathogens; IgG, IgD and IgE act on their own as monomers, which means one antibody binds to only one antigen (a pathogen may have many antigens), IgA works in couples (dimers) at respiratory, intestinal, and urogenital surfaces, while the IgM, attacks a pathogen as a polymer of five individual IgM molecules (pentameter) (Fig. 6.5).

But what happens after the liaison between the antigen and antibody has occurred? The protection mechanisms that follow can be different: the simplest is the neutralization, by which the antibody blocks vital parts of the cell or the virus making their attack unsuccessful. The antibodies can also aggregate and stick to foreign cells (e.g., bacteria and tumor cells) and proteins, which are later eaten by the macrophages in the blood or in the tissues.

The Complement System

Complement is a complex mechanism made up of a series of proteins acting as enzymes and it works by (a) attracting immune cells towards bacteria, (b) making the pathogens tastier for macrophages and neutrophils and, (c) piercing the cell

The importance of the Complement system

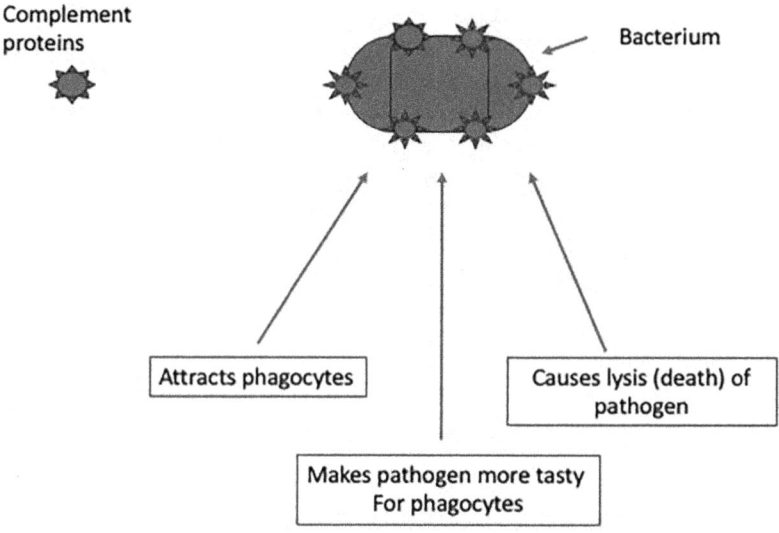

Fig. 6.6 The complement system: complement proteins attach to pathogens and have three main functions. (**a**) It sends out a signal that attracts phagocytes; (**b**) makes the pathogen more tasty for phagocytes; (**c**) kills the pathogen through lysis* (breaking it open)

membranes of pathogens (Fig. 6.6). The complement system is like a cascade of enzymes that results in perforating the pathogen and making it easy prey for the macrophages.

The complement system also contributes to the inflammatory response.

Inflammation

Inflammation is the body's process that fights against harmful things like infections, injuries, tumors and toxins, to heal itself. This protective response is generated by blood cells, blood vessels, and soluble mediators (such as cytokines*, especially interferons, and interleukins). Cytokines are chemical mediators released by different cells. The "acute inflammatory response" is meant to localize and eliminate pathogens so that tissues can regenerate and heal. Acute inflammation is initially localized and visually characterized by swelling (in Latin, tumor), redness (rubor) and pain (in Latin, dolor), an increase in temperature (calor), and subsequently, could bring about the impairment of the function of the involved tissues or organs.

The *Kinin System* also participates in inflammation. Kinins are responsible for pain, along with substances active in the blood vessels such as histamine and serotonin mediators. In essence, (acute) inflammation is a complex and broadly acting mechanism of the innate immune response that has the role of limiting, protecting, and repairing an affected or damaged area. However, if the cause of the inflammation persists, it becomes chronic and if is very strong, it can spread throughout the entire body.

Inflammation is named differently depending on the organ where it develops: appendix = appendicitis, pancreas = pancreatitis, peritoneum = peritonitis, myocardium = myocarditis, bronchi = bronchitis, and so on. Chronic inflammation usually involves lymphocytes (of the acquired immune system) as well as the innate system and may cause a variety of complications: thrombosis, metabolic syndrome, atherosclerosis, liver disease, neurological disorders, obesity, and other issues.

Chapter 7
Hematology and Immunology

The late nineteenth century and the beginning of the twentieth century was an important time for science and particularly for discovering the fundamental aspects of hematology and immunology.

Paul Ehrlich's pioneering work on blood cells using various dyes identified many of the blood cells that we subsequently know are important cells in the immune system. At around the same time, Iiya Metchnikoff was discovering phagocytosis. He was carrying out experiments using starfish larvae and observed that when foreign particles, such as thorns or tiny splinters, were introduced into these organisms, specialized cells, which he termed "phagocytes," would migrate to the site of injury and engulf and destroy the foreign material through a process he called "phagocytosis." He also observed that this was the process by which certain white blood cells engulf and destroy pathogens. These were some of the white blood cells that Ehrlich had recently identified by their staining characteristics.

Meanwhile, Emil von Behring and Shibasaburo Kitasato, working independently carried out experiments in which they showed that serum from animals previously exposed to certain diseases could confer immunity to other animals when injected. They termed the substance responsible for this immunity "antitoxin," which we now know as antibodies. They went on to study diphtheria and anti-diphtheria toxins for which von Behring received the first Nobel Prize in Physiology and Medicine in 1901.

Following the discovery of antibodies, Ehrlich proposed that cells possess specific receptor sites, which he referred to as "side chains," on their surface. These receptor sites are capable of binding to specific foreign substances called antigens. He also compared the interaction between antigens and antibodies to a lock-and-key mechanism. According to his theory, each antigen has a unique shape that corresponds to the shape of specific receptor sites on immune cells.

His theory provided a framework for understanding the specificity of immune responses and his concept of "horror autotoxicus" (fear of self-toxicity) suggested that the body's immune system could distinguish between self and non-self.

G. Mariani et al., *Blood: The Science, History, and Mysteries of Life's Vital Flow*, https://doi.org/10.1007/978-3-031-92481-1_7

Metchnikoff's research on phagocytosis and Ehrlich's 'side chain theory' laid the groundwork for our understanding of the cellular components of the immune system and the specificity of antibodies and earned them the Nobel Prize in Physiology and Medicine in 1908.

So, these early scientific discoveries led to the foundation for modern immunology and significantly influenced subsequent research in the field.

Subsequently, many other significant discoveries relating to hematology and immunology were made.

In the early twentieth century Landsteiner discovered red cell blood types (groups) crucial for understanding immune reactions and transplantation compatibility. He received the Nobel Prize for Physiology or Medicine in 1930.

There was much progress in Immunology in the late twentieth century. The concept of cellular immunity*, which involves the direct action of immune cells against infected or abnormal cells, was further developed by researchers Frank Macfarlane Burnet and Peter Medawar. They also developed the concept of acquired 'immunological tolerance' (this is why our immune systems don't normally attack our own tissues). For this they were awarded the Nobel Prize for Physiology and Medicine in 1960.

The structure of antibodies, elucidated by Michael Heidelberger and Linus Pauling, provided insights as to how antibodies interact with antigens. This was at a time when antibodies were identified as being in the globulins fraction of plasma. Rodney Porter and Gerry Edelman used enzymes to split IgG antibody molecules into their heavy and light chains (Fig. 6.5). They identified the part of the molecule that was specific and that part that had biological function. For this, Porter and Edelman received the Nobel Prize in Physiology or Medicine in 1972.

In 1959 Jim Gowans showed that lymphocytes migrate from blood to lymph and back again and in the 1960s it was shown that there were two types (classes) of lymphocytes with different functions, T (thymus derived), and B (bursa derived). Robert Good and Max Cooper working in a chicken model found that the Bursa of Fabricius was responsible for antibody production and that cells required an intact thymus for producing delayed-type hypersensitivity (a cellular response).

Towards the late part of the twentieth century, the major histocompatibility complex (MHC) was discovered, and its role in antigen presentation, by researchers including George Snell and Jean Dausset, advanced understanding of immune responses and transplantation immunology. For these findings, Snell, Dausset and Baruj Benacerraf received the Nobel Prize in Physiology and Medicine in 1980.

The clonal selection theory proposed by Frank Macfarlane Burnet, and David Talmage in the mid-twentieth century provided a comprehensive framework for understanding how the immune system recognizes and responds to antigens.

Fig. 7.1 Relationship between hematology and immunology. There is a great deal of overlap between the two sciences

Hematology is about one third Immunology

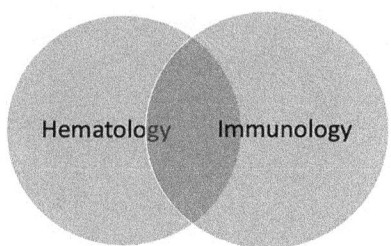

This theory was extended by Neils Jerne and he shared the Nobel Prize in Physiology and Medicine in 1984 with Georges J. F. Köhler and César Milstein "for theories concerning the specificity in development and control of the immune system and the discovery of the principle for production of monoclonal antibodies".

This latter finding initiated the era of immunotherapy*, now a major tool in the treatment of cancer and autoimmune diseases (see Chap. 15).

As you see from the information just given in this sub-chapter and in other places in the book, Immunology and Hematology are intimately linked with Hematology overlapping with Immunology by about a third (Fig. 7.1).

Chapter 8
Where Blood Is Made, the Bone Marrow

At the beginning, the cells studied were those in the peripheral blood, easily obtainable from peripheral veins. We now know that cells of the blood originate from the bone marrow, a relatively recent discovery. Since the marrow is hidden in the bones and its presence is elusive, Galenus, Aristotle, and Hippocrates thought that this mushy tissue of the bones was a waste product, resulting from bone renewal. It was only at the end of the nineteenth century that the studies by Neumann, Bizzozzero and Osler demonstrated that the marrow was the site of blood production. By using the Ehrich's dyes, it became possible to study the morphology and function of this elusive tissue. These studies, which provided a lot of the information for approximately a century, now appear redundant due to the advances in molecular and cell biology. In fact, new technologies allow precise information on blood cells and their precursors without the need to examine them under a microscope.

At any rate, at the beginning of the twentieth century, Ehrlich hypothesized that there were interactions between cells as well as hierarchies among the different cell lineages. But it was only with the studies of Adolfo Ferrata, one of the founders of Hematology, we could conclude that the cell from which the blood originates is not a lymphocyte (although it look like one), but is a totipotent stem cell. Ferrata's vision was correct: the cell that he called hemocytoblast would later be named Stem Cell.

A few primitive stem cells in our mothers' womb can produce all the tissues and organs of our bodies, up to and through adulthood. The stem cells in a healthy adult keep us alive by producing and renewing the blood and immune system cells every day. In humans, the hematopoietic (from Greek, aema = blood, poiesis = production) and the immune systems originate in the marrow, again showing the overlap of Hematology and Immunology. It is for this reason that marrow, circulating blood, and the immune system can together be considered as an organ, with the function of protecting and keeping us alive.

The hematopoietic bone marrow produces the astonishing amount of 500 billion (500×10^9) mature cells every day. The close collaboration between immune cell

G. Mariani et al., *Blood: The Science, History, and Mysteries of Life's Vital Flow*, https://doi.org/10.1007/978-3-031-92481-1_8

production and blood cell production is only found in more complex organisms and, thus, in human beings. Why does the marrow appear either yellow or red? The 'active' marrow is red because it produces large amounts of hemoglobin, while the yellow marrow is 'inactive', hidden in a sea of fat cells, that can shift to the red one if needed (for example, to deal with an infection or a hemorrhage).

What is a 'Stem Cell"? A Stem Cell is the only cell capable of self-replication and able to develop into different types of cells which progressively become mature cells (differentiation). Self-replication is required to maintain a stable reservoir of stem cells in the body. However, from the embryo to adulthood, stem cells change their functional potential.

In simple terms, stem cells are rather like the fertilized egg (zygote), which contains the genetic information to develop into any cell of the body. A haemopoietic stem cell (HSC) was once thought to just give rise to different blood cells, but this dogma is changing with more and more data suggesting that it can give rise to other cells in the body. In fact, a small number of stem cells is present in the various tissues of the body with the aim of replacing local cells that have died and to repair injured tissues.

The stem cells in the marrow and the other tissues are present for the entire life of an individual, but their numbers progressively decrease with age. Perhaps the process of getting old is related to this reduction. The identification of stem cells has triggered an appetite for research and for their use in congenital as well as acquired diseases (Alzheimer's, Parkinsons'). Stem cell manipulation is not easy and requires the support of complex technological facilities (stem cell factories). Moreover, there are ethical issues that need to be considered. To date, some living animals have been cloned* from stem cells, including the carp, cattle, rabbits, dogs, cats, pigs, sheep, and macaques. It is reasonable to ask: why are stem cells specialized in the particular tissues where they reside? There is scientific evidence indicating that their differentiation potential is linked to the specific microenvironment present in each tissue. This is likely to be due to specific chemicals like cytokines and the interaction of the stem cells with each other and with the stromal cells. However, the SC specialization varies depending on the microenvironment.

Adult stem cells (number-plated CD34) produce impressive amounts of blood and immune system components every hour and every day of our lives. How is this huge production of different types of cells (lineages) organized? The marrow stem cells give rise to the production of the different cellular lineages identified by the suffix-poiesis (from the Greek produce: for example, erythro<u>poiesis</u>, granulo<u>poiesis</u> and so on). Each cellular lineage is composed of intermediate mother cells which, through maturation and differentiation, give rise to daughter cells until they mature into specialized cells (e.g. monos, NeutroPhils). The single precursors of the different hematopoietic lineages are identified with the suffix 'blast': the precursors of the red cells are erythro<u>blasts</u>, those of lymphocytes are called lympho<u>blasts</u>, those of granulocytes are called granulo<u>blasts</u>, and of monocytes mono<u>blasts</u>; the only exception is with the platelets, their precursors being megakaryoblasts and megakaryocytes.

In adulthood, the marrow represents 4% of the body mass (between 2.5 and 3 kg), a lot if compared with the liver (about 2.45 kg), the brain a little more than 2%, both lungs 2%, while the heart and the kidneys are only 0.5% each. In the adult, the marrow resides in the flat bones (sternum, ribs, pelvic bones, and cranium), and in the terminal parts of long bones [epiphyses].

The production of blood cells is quite a complex process. Recently, a new model was proposed based on two assumptions. Firstly, there is a daily production of around 500 billion cells, and secondly, there is a population of around 80 million stem cells, of which only 10% are active. This means that there are eight million 'subunits' of marrow, each producing 50–70,000 mature cells and each having its anatomical niche. Spatially, the progenitors start developing in the niche* and continue their development moving towards the surface of the sinusoids (capillaries of the marrow) where the mature cells are released. This model helps us to understand the passage of so many cells into the blood. It is like a comb, with the teeth turned towards the niches (Fig. 8.1).

The cell precursors push the mature cells towards the capillaries (Fig. 8.1), which, in turn, converge into the sinusoids and then into the general circulation. The cells that get into the circulation are of many types and quantities, but the numbers of circulating blood cells need to be kept stable. 40% of the total marrow output is red blood cells, 30% platelets and 20% granulocytes. This implies the presence of a precisely regulated system (Fig. 8.2). The functions and characteristics of the marrow are summarized in Table 8.1.

And the lymphocytes in the marrow? They are quite numerous (12–16%) in adulthood and the vast majority are identifiable as B lymphocytes. Once produced, some lymphocyte precursors migrate via the bloodstream into the thymus where they develop into specialized T lymphocytes. However, little is known about the lymphoid lineage of the marrow and the mechanism that selects these precursor T lymphocytes to migrate to the thymus.

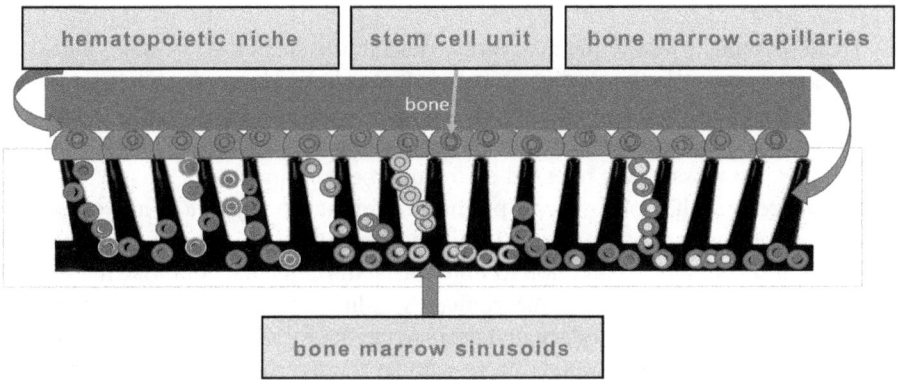

Fig. 8.1 The marrow vascular tree. Schematic representation of the developmental sequence and output of blood cells in the bone marrow. The different colored cells indicate the different cell lineages

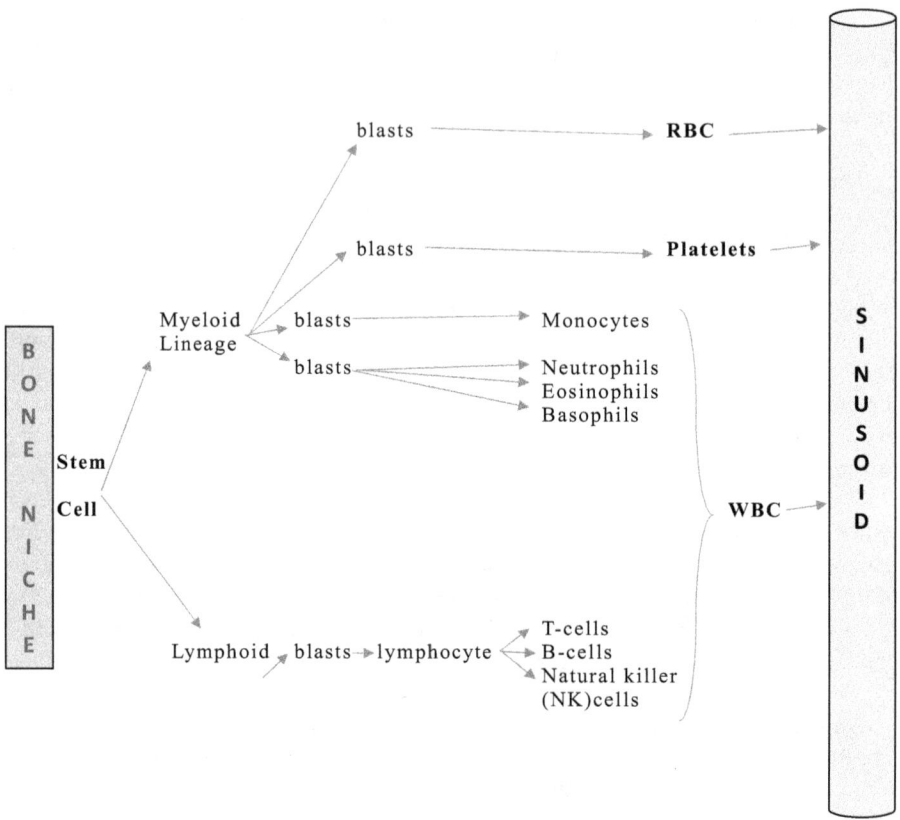

Fig. 8.2 Bone marrow: flow-chart of the blood cell production. The stem cells give rise to two lineages—myeloid and lymphoid. The myeloid lineage through blasts produces RBCs, platelets, and all the white blood cells (monocytes, neutrophils eosinophils, and basophils) except lymphocytes that are produced within the lymphoid lineage. T, B and NK* cells

The environment where the marrow carries out this amazing job is unique since delicate interactions between diverse cells are required. The marrow lies on a web of loose semi-fluid tissue called stroma composed of fibers, cells, and interstitial fluids that, together, constitute the 'microenvironment'. Interactions between cells occur thanks to messangers released by the microenvironment.

Stroma cells in the bone marrow produce different growth factors and other factors that are necessary for the specific activation and differentiation of the stem cells and the cell precursors. In addition to fibroblasts, the cells that comprise the stroma in individual 'niches 'include macrophages, adipocytes (fat cells), osteoblasts, osteoclasts (the cells that produce and destroy the bone), and endothelial cells.

For example, if we look at the marrow under the microscope, we can see a distinct morphological structure called an Erythroblastic island. This is characterized by a cellular aggregate consisting of a central MacroPhage (which is called a Nurse Cell), surrounded by red blood cell precursors (Fig. 8.3). This MacroPhage contains

Table 8.1 Summary of bone marrow functions and characteristics

Overall mass	4% of the body weight (2.5–3 kg)
Mature cell production and release into the circulation	5 billions cells/day
Total stem cell content	80 millions
Active stem cells	10%: 8 millions
Marrow units	8 millions
Production of cells/unit/day	60–70,000
Lineage production	40% RBC 30% Platelets 20% Granulocytes
Proportion of marrow lineages and cells	Granuloblasts 55–60% Erythroblasts 20–25% Lymphocytes 12–16% Plasma cells 1–2% Monocytes & macrophages 0.5–2% Megakaryocytes 0.5–1%
Marrow sinusoid density	25,000/mm^3

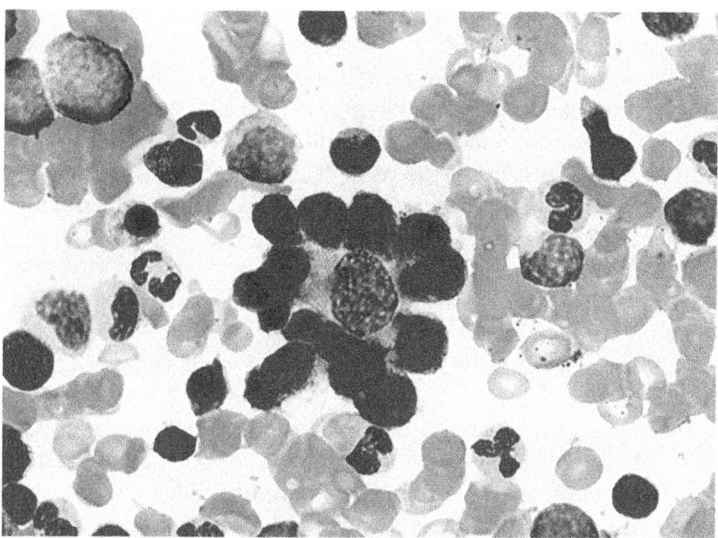

Fig. 8.3 The Erythroblastic island. Iron is transferred from a macrophage (red) surrounded by the red cell precursors (blue)

iron granules, which are transferred to the red blood cell precursors so that hemo-globin production can be completed.

Other important interactions are those that occur between stroma cells and stem cells in the niche: the osteoblasts (cells that produce the bone tissue) are essential for stem cell activation whilst osteoclasts (the cells that promote the reabsorption of bone tissue) depress stem cell function. There is relatively little knowledge about the many and complex interactions between the marrow cells in terms of dynamism:

the niches can regress, disappear, and new ones can form. This phenomenon is the basis for the expansion/regression of marrow.

The marrow also receives signals from chemical messengers (cytokines*) produced by various organs in the body, which can stimulate or depress its activity. A few are 'specific' for a certain lineage, but others have a larger activity spectrum.

There are many of these cytokines (from the Greek cyto = cell and kinesis = movement) or 'growth factors'*. Many of these have now been produced artificially from their genes. The first to be identified was the now-famous erythropoietin (EPO), which stimulates the erythroblasts to produce red blood cells. Other cytokines include GM-CSF (Granulocyte-Monocyte-Colony Stimulating Factor which stimulates the Phil and Mono lineages), M-CSF (Monocyte-CSF, which stimulates the Mono precursors), G-CSF (which stimulates the Phil lineage), interleukin-3 (IL-3, broad spectrum stimulating), interleukin 5 (IL-5, the regulator of the eosinophil lineage), Stem Cell Factor (SCF, stimulating among other things the self-maintenance of the stem cells) and thrombopoietin (TPO, stimulating the production of platelets). However, most of these growth factors have a wide or very wide activity spectrum.

Most of these substances are produced by tissues/organs external to the marrow: EPO is mainly produced by the kidney, GM-CSF by fibroblasts (stromal cells in the marrow or elsewhere), and endothelial cells in various organs (lungs, muscle, etc.), M-SCF also by fibroblasts, IL-3 from some lymphocytes, and TPO from the liver. The target cells of these cytokines have specific sensors (receptors) on their surface, resulting in a series of reactions, the most relevant leading to the increase in cell survival and proliferation, or to the performance of specific functions, as protein production or Apoptosis* (programmed cell death).

Cytokines can work across short distances as in the marrow, or like EPO in the entire body, like hormones. Regarding clinical use, G-CSF is used to increase the number of stem cells in the blood before collection for bone marrow transplantation (See Chap. 15). However, EPO is by far the most frequently used cytokine in clinical practice. Its most accredited use is for the treatment of anemia in patients with renal diseases (inflamed kidneys no longer produce EPO) or in patients with malignancies involving the marrow. At any rate, hormones like cortisone and thyroid hormones have a strong impact on the marrow, to mention but a few.

We think it is interesting to remember how EPO has become notorious since being used for doping in athletes (dope: illegal drug use). EPO, by increasing the quantity of hemoglobin in the blood, leads to a significant increase in an athlete's aerobic capacity (the capacity to keep up a medium/fast rhythm for a fixed time).

The athlete's aerobic capacity (called VO_2Max the highest amount of oxygen used in a unit of time to make movements) increases in parallel with hemoglobin levels.

The first athlete identified to have taken EPO was the French cyclist Erwann Mentheour during the Tour de France in 1997. Another athlete who was found positive in an antidoping test was the swede Niklas Axelsson, who won the Tour in 2000. The first athlete who died because of doping was a 19-year-old Russian hockey player, Alexei Cherepanov, the dose he was using was very high. Over time, various athletes have been accused of having taken doping substances in numerous sports, both during the Olympic Games and in other events. In many cases, the National and International Sports Federations were involved in these scandals since, frequently, they were protecting the athletes. Also, the cyclist Lance Armstrong was accused of taking doping substances and EPO during his career and this led to the invalidation of his seven victories in the Tour de France.

EPO has also been used in sports where anaerobic activities predominate, such as boxing: two boxers of the UFL (Ultimate Fighter Championship) were found to be positive for EPO. We have a suspicion that tennis players take it during tournaments. EPO can help you when you are in the fifth set and you have played for four and a half hours! When non-doped players have an unmet oxygen requirement, the doped ones are still able to play and ultimately win. The problem with EPO is that while there are positive effects on the VO_2Max lasting a couple of weeks, there is no trace of this substance in the blood or urine after 36–48 hours. According to Martha Brant's inquiry published in Newsweek, the use of EPO has killed at least 18 Dutch and Belgian cyclists since 1987.

Beyond its unquestionable illegal use in sports, there are several hazards for those who take it even if it does not result in complications. EPO increases the red blood cell number (up to 1.5–2 million), causing an increase in blood viscosity. In an athlete taking EPO, the speed of circulating blood increases rapidly, but at the end of the physical activity, blood hyperviscosity takes over worsened by dehydration, and therefore the blood pressure increases and the heart activity is surcharged.

Other drugs that are taken for performance enhancement, like testosterone and growth hormone increase muscular mass, and so are taken by athletes, especially for bodybuilding. However, these drugs also increase EPO's endogenous production, creating harmful synergistic effects. Side effects are absent when EPO is used as a support treatment for cancer or renal disease.

Strangely enough, sporting organizations do not appear to propose post-mortem investigations in the case of suspicious deaths due to doping!

Chapter 9
How Blood Gets Around the Body

At this point, we need to understand how arterial blood, venous blood and lymph differ in terms of patterns of flow and functions.

The main functions of blood are:

- Transport of Oxygen and Nutrients: oxygenated blood is pumped from the lungs to the rest of the body and returns deoxygenated to the lungs for a new oxygenation. It also delivers essential nutrients from the digestive system to the cells of the body.
- Waste Product Removal: Blood carries waste products, such as carbon dioxide and urea, from the cells to the lungs and kidneys for excretion. This helps maintain a clean and balanced internal environment.
- Regulation of Body Temperature: The flow of blood helps to regulate body temperature by distributing heat throughout the body. And, when the body needs to release excess heat, blood vessels near the skin surface dilate, allowing more blood to flow through them and release heat.
- Hormone Distribution: These are chemical messengers released by certain glands and carried by the blood to target organs and tissues.
- Immune System Function: Blood contains some cells of the immune system and other components of the immune system that help to protect the body against infections and diseases.
- Hemostasis: This is the mechanism by which blood changes from a fluid to a gel, contributing to stop blood losses.
- Maintaining Homeostasis: The circulation of blood by the heart helps maintain homeostasis by balancing the pH levels, ion concentrations, and fluid volumes in the different parts of the body.

The story about blood circulation started with William Harvey (who graduated in Medicine at the University of Padua in the early seventeenth century). When returned to England, he conducted several experiments and concluded that blood is pushed by the heart into the arteries and returns to the heart through the veins. The

G. Mariani et al., *Blood: The Science, History, and Mysteries of Life's Vital Flow*, https://doi.org/10.1007/978-3-031-92481-1_9

heart was considered to be like a sort of mechanical pump and not the location of the soul, as previously believed.

He could not understand the mechanism of blood oxygenation, since oxygen had not yet been discovered and was surprised when he did not find air in the pulmonary vein, the vessel that connects the lungs to the left part of the heart. Only with the work of the French scientist Antoine Lavoisier, at the end of the 1700s, oxygen and its role in respiration were discovered. Lavoisier gave the elements he discovered the names of oxygen (O_2) and hydrogen (H). After Harvey, it became clear that arteries and veins have different characteristics (as is the case for lymphatics). The tubes containing the blood or the lymph are found all over the body and are generically called 'vessels' (blood vessels or lymphatic vessels); all the vessels together are referred to as the circulatory tree. External sheaths of either smooth muscle or elastic fibers confer elasticity and resistance to the vessels (i.e. capillary artery, vein, and ducts), features that are required for their function. Circulation of body fluids not only involves the transport of oxygen, carbon dioxide, nutrients, waste, cells, and proteins that defend our body, but also maintains the balance between the various compartments and ultimately ensures the integrity of the vascular tree. Moreover, hormones produced by the various endocrine glands (for example, thyroid, pituitary, adrenal, and pineal glands) can reach their target organs via blood circulation.

Finally, fluid exchanges are so well regulated that the volume of blood, lymph, and extracellular fluids remains constant. Blood is pushed into the vascular tree from the heart where it circulates under various pressures: in the arteries, it has a pressure of 120 mmHg which then decreases to 2–3 mmHg when it returns to the right atrium of the heart; the pressure then increases to 15–20 mmHg in the lungs, decreases again to 3 mmHg in the left atrium and finally returns to 120 mmHg in the aorta. Arteries are so resistant and elastic that they can tolerate over 200 mmHg of pressure due to their abundant elastic fibers. The large and medium-sized arteries pulsate because blood is pushed intermittently by the heart's contractions. Also, due to the elastic fibers, the blood flow becomes continuous in the vessels distant from the heart (as is the case of arterioles, capillaries, and veins). All the capillaries have a surface area greater than 1000 times that of the aorta, and this is the reason why blood loses speed.

At rest and under normal conditions, blood is distributed to the various organs in different quantities.

Of the five liters of blood pumped by the heart every minute, 21% enter the muscles, 20% the kidneys, 20% the gastrointestinal system, 14% the brain, 14% the bones and the skin, 7% the liver, and 4% the heart vessels.

What are the reasons for this diverse distribution of blood? The first is related to the anatomy: the aorta (starting from the left ventricle) is like a motorway and the exits are of different sizes and therefore, the amount of blood that leaves the aorta depends on each vessel's diameter. For example, renal arteries are large, but the coronaries and the intercostal arteries are small. Moreover, peripheral arteries, i.e. the arterioles (2–3 mm in diameter) are provided with muscles that work as valves that regulate the quantity of blood that can pass into different anatomical sites; this mechanism is under the control of the Involuntary Nervous System (also called the sympathetic nervous system). This is the distribution of blood at rest. However, the circulation is organized in a way that different organs and tissues, depending on their immediate needs may receive increased or decreased amounts of blood.

For example, during your run in the park, blood is pumped mainly to the muscles, heart, and lungs, while during digestion the stomach and bowel are prioritized; skin can receive a lot of blood if exposed to the sun or if the body temperature is elevated (to allow heat dispersion) and so on.

In the veins, the speed of blood increases from the periphery towards the heart thanks to the muscle fibres present in the vessel wall (under the control of the involuntary musculature). Moreover, a huge help to the blood flow in the veins is provided by the muscles of the lower limbs, which surround and compress the deep veins. Furthermore, veins and lymphatic trunks possess valves that let the blood/lymph flow in one direction only. Veins have walls that are thinner than the arteries (average ratio of thickness/diameter 1/40 compared to 1/10): this explains the fragility of the veins when the internal pressure increases (Table 9.1).

An important question is: how long does it take for a single blood cell to complete the circuit from the heart, back to the heart? It depends on the route that the blood takes which can be very variable. However, we can estimate the time required on the basis that the heart pumps about 7100 liters of blood over 24 h, which is 4.9 liters of blood a minute (roughly the total volume of blood). Thus, one minute is necessary for the blood to make the complete tour of the circulatory tree. This means that blood circulates about 1500 times over 24 h. An echocardiogram (echography of the heart) can precisely measure the amount of blood pushed by the heart into the aorta at each single heartbeat (or 'systole'); thus, considering the number of beats over time, the calculation can be easily done.

There is an important aspect regarding the interactions between vessel walls and blood. No matter what they are, all vessels (arteries, capillaries, lymphatics, and veins) are covered by flat cells (endothelial cells) that link up to form a continuous floor over which the blood flows. Endothelial cells have different functional characteristics depending on which organ they are in. For example, in the kidney glomerulus, the endothelium filters the fluids and selects the dissolved salts for removal in the urine, but in the marrow, the mature cells continue to pass into the blood. Moreover, endothelial cells contribute (through substances they secrete) to the dilation and contraction of the vessels, regulating, in this way, the hemostasis and the coagulation mechanisms (which prevents hemorrhage). Endothelial cells also recruit neutrophils through the release of specific substances and contribute to hormone trafficking. Thus, this extensive floor of cells making up the endothelium (some consider it like an organ), has metabolic functions, can sense signals coming from the blood and react to them accordingly. The endothelium of the heart is called the endocardium.

****

Table 9.1 Details of the circulatory tree

Parameter	Measure	Note
Total length of the circulatory tree	80.000–150.000 km	Arteries + veins + capillaries
Maximum artery diameter	Circa 4 cm	Ascending aorta
Average artery diameter	4 mm	
Average artery wall thickness	1 mm	
Maximum vein diameter	3 cm	Superior Vena Cava
	3.3 cm	Inferior Vena Cava
Average vein diameter	5 mm	
Average vein wall thickness	0.5 mm	
Average capillary diameter	8 µm	
Average capillary wall thickness	0.5 µm	
Total fluid volume	16 litri	Blood + extracellular fluids + Lymph
Total blood volume*	Man 4.8954 liters	Height 175 cm, weight 75 kg
	Female 4.1694 liters	Height 165 cm, weight 60 kg
Total plasma volume	Man 2.300 litri	Mean haematocrit 47%
	Woman 1.751 liters	Mean haematocrit 42%
Lymph volume	0.3 liters	
Arterial blood pressure	120 – 80 b mmHg	Systole – diastole
Pulmonary blood pressure	25–12 mmHg	Diastole – systole
Capillary pressure	10–20 mmHg	
Venous pressure	2–3 mmHg	Central
Venous pressure	3–5 mmHg	Abdominal
Venous pressure	8–10 mmHg	Inguinal
Maximal pressure exerted by the heart	130 cm/s (4.68 km/h)	Left ventricle
Arterial blood speed	45–50 cm/s (1.6–1.8 km/h)	Large vessels
Venous blood speed	20–45 cm/s (0.7–1.6 km/h)	
Speed of capillary blood and lymph	0.03–0.07 cm/s (1.1–2.5 m/h)	
Snail speed for comparison	0.13 cm/s (4.7 m/h)	

The liquids (fluids) of the body are categorized into two main compartments, the intracellular—maintained within cells, and the extracellular compartment comprising the Plasma (in the arteries and veins), the Lymph (in the lymphatic vessels), the Cerebrospinal fluid (in the central nervous system), and the Interstitial fluid that supplies all the cells. The interstitial fluid (that fills the spaces between the cells) contains some proteins and a few cells and supplies the cells and the tissues by diffusion: if these fluids are in excess, they cause Edema, and if they lack cause Dehydration.

The Role of the Lymphatic System

The Lymph circulates inside the lymphatic vessels. The name derives from the Latin Goddess that protected font water, Lymfa. It contains mineral salts, products of metabolism, and lymphocytes of the adaptive immune system. Bacteria, viruses, foreign substances, and also tumor cells can all get into the lymph which carries them to the lymphatic organs where are processed by the body's defense mechanisms. Lymphatic circulation is a widespread part of the circulatory system. It passes through the tissues and organs of the immune system and then back to the bloodstream. This connection between tissues, organs of the immune system and blood allows us to understand the complexity and the importance of the lymphatic system.

During the evolution from unicellular to multicellular organisms, interstitial fluid served to connect the various cells and tissues and we can imagine this being similar in function to the lymph. The appearance of the lymph varies according to the organ/tissue of origin: generally, it has a pale yellowish color that doesn't differ from that of plasma. Conversely, the lymph that drains the intestinal lymphatic system is milky (rich in fat drops) as it is released into the general lymphatic circulation and then into the blood. A specific feature of lymph is that it contains no 'sticky' proteins (the correct term is adhesive: fibrinogen, von Willebrand), or platelets. This prevents lymph from 'clotting' even though it has a very slow flow. What's more, the lymph that enters the lymphatic organs e.g. lymph nodes (afferent lymph) contains few lymphocytes, whereas the lymph leaving the lymphatic organs (efferent lymph) contains so many lymphocytes that it might be considered to be a liquid lymphatic tissue.

But let's now try to understand how lymphatic circulation works. Its most obvious role is to return the fluids that have left the blood system, back into the blood circulation. The interstitial fluid that has bathed the tissues returns in the same amount but is enriched with the products of the tissue metabolism together with specialized cells of the immune system. Drainage of fluids from different parts of the body occurs through the lymph circulatory system; just imagine the lymph capillary web as being like a spider web that channels the new 'lymph' towards the center of the web. The lymph nodes at the center of this spider's web, filter the lymph. These webs are present all over the body except in the hematopoietic marrow, the nervous system, and in the skin. From the lymph nodes, the lymph is conveyed into larger and larger lymphatic vessels until it reaches the large lymphatic ducts, of which there are two: the Right one which drains the lymph from the right-hand upper side of the body and the Thoracic duct that drains the rest of the body. The ducts pour the lymph into the deep venous system of the shoulder on the right and left sides. Let's remember that the lymph from the Thoracic duct is milky due to it being rich in fats absorbed by the bowel. Hence, the lymph mixes with the venous blood and then reaches the right side of the heart.

But how does this small amount of fluid (only 1/3 of liter) move through the lymph vessels? Firstly, a minimum hydrostatic pressure is enough to push it into the lymphatic vessels. Other help is provided by the smooth (involuntary) musculature present in the walls of the capillaries and the lymphatic vessels, but the main push is generated by the contraction of voluntary muscles such as the quadriceps and calf muscles in the leg. Finally, the presence of valves keeps the lymph flowing only in the direction towards the heart.

After birth, the immune system develops and becomes functional in the Lymphoid Organs, which are of two types: the Primary and the Secondary (Table 9.2). Essentially, the primary organs produce the lymphoid cells while the secondary (which are mainly connected with the lymphatic vessels), modify them and contribute to their maturation so that they can attack foreign invaders (bacteria, viruses etc.) as part of the immune response.

In adulthood, the primary lymphoid organs are the bone marrow and the thymus, but during fetal life, it is the liver. The thymus is a small organ (but larger in a newborn child) that is located posteriorly and superiorly to the heart. All the lymphocytes originate from stem cells in the marrow through a process called "lymphopoiesis", which gives rise to two main tribes of lymphocytes: "B" lymphocytes develop directly from stem cells in the Bone Marrow and "T" lymphocytes from T cell progenitor cells that migrate from the bone marrow via the circulation and continue their development in the Thymus (Chap. 6). Both B cells and T cells migrate into the secondary lymphoid organs to mature and carry out their functions. The secondary lymphoid/lymphatic organs include (Table 9.2) (a) the lymph nodes, small, kidney-shaped organelles, with a diameter of about one centimeter. Around 500–600 lymph nodes are located along the lymphatic vessels and are heavily grouped at the center of the lymphatic webs; and (b) the spleen (an abdominal organ with a longitudinal diameter of 10 cm). From a functional point of view, this is like a large lymph node that filters the blood but not the lymph. Finally, there are (c) the aggregates of lymphoid tissue, which are in the mucosal walls of the digestive, pulmonary, and urogenital tracts. Secondary lymphoid aggregates are also present in the tonsils and the tubes of the female reproductive system.

Table 9.2 Organs/tissues of the immune system

Organ	Site
Bone marrow	Bones (P)
Spleen	Abdomen, left hypochondrium (S)
Thymus	Thorax, behind the sternum (P)
Lymph nodes	Axilla, neck, abdomen, groin (S)
Tonsils & adenoids	Naso-pharyngeal cavity (S)
Payer's patches	Small bowel (S)
Mucosal-associated lymphoid tissue	Mucous membranes (S)
Skin-associated lymphoid tissue	In the dermis (S)
Thoracic duct	Upper abdomen and thorax
Appendix	Abdomen, lower right side (S)

P = primary, S = secondary
P, primary organs: where the lymphocytes are produced; S, secondary organs/tissues: where the lymphocytes recognize and respond to microbial invaders

The maturation and function of lymphocytes depend on which tribe they belong to. The T lymphocytes are selected in the thymus based on their skills of recognizing antigens (foreign substances, bacteria, and viruses) but not to react against the body's antigens. Only 5% of T lymphocytes leave the thymus as mature T lymphocytes, the remaining 95% die through a process called 'apoptosis' (programmed cell death). The thymus is a very active organ until adolescence and then gradually shrinks with age.

The T lymphocytes that leave the thymus are heterogeneous in their function, they circulate everywhere in the body and colonize the secondary lymphatic organs where interact with B lymphocytes. Lymphocytes enter the lymphoid organs and tissues through specialized venules and pass out via the efferent lymphatic vessels that push the lymph into the ducts and, finally, into the bloodstream (see above).

In the lymphoid tissues, mature T and B lymphocytes interact with foreign invaders (bacteria, viruses, etc.), and start the process of antibody production, or become 'memory' cells. The B lymphocytes may differentiate into plasma cells (the 'antibody factories'), cells that produce large quantities of the same antibody. The "memory B lymphocytes" represent a sort of historical archive of the foreign invaders that the body has been exposed to over time.

Part III
Disorders of the Blood

Chapter 10
Not Having Enough Hemoglobin: Anemia

Anemia Due to Loss of Iron

The mechanism that prevents blood from coming out of the circulatory tree is complex and many events can alter it. When this mechanism fails, the loss of a large quantity of blood (e.g. in a stomach ulcer), or a frequent small quantity of blood (e.g. some tumors or hemorrhoids) can occur. In any case, if significant quantities of iron are lost, this affects blood production.

Hemoglobin is an iron-containing protein, a main constituent of red blood cells (RBC): it is the protein that allows us to breathe! The marrow precursors of RBC cannot produce hemoglobin if no iron is available. When the hemoglobin levels decrease, this leads to the most common and well-known consequence of anemia, Fatigue (doctors call it asthenia = loss of strength), which is roughly proportional to the reduction in the amount of hemoglobin. However, when the process is insidious (as it is often seen in iron deficiency caused by heavy periods), the tolerance to fatigue is higher.

Lack of iron is the most common dietary deficiency in the world: it affects about 60% of children and women in developing countries, and 50% of these individuals suffer from anemia-related symptoms. We are talking about over one billion people! On the other hand, in developed countries, only 10–20% of women suffer from anemia. But, if we focus on pregnant women, the prevalence of iron deficiency is indeed higher. But why is there such a delicate balance between iron metabolism and anemia? Why is iron deficiency so prevalent in women?

The quantity of iron in the entire body is only 4 g in men and 3.2 in women and children (Fig. 10.1). Of this, 2/3rd is part of the hemoglobin (2.6 g in men, 2.1 g in women, 2 g in children), and the remaining 1/3rd is stored in the 'deposits' (600–1000 mg in men, 200–400 mg in women 100–200 mg in children). Iron is stored mainly in the liver and the muscles. Figure 10.2 shows the mechanism of iron accumulation.

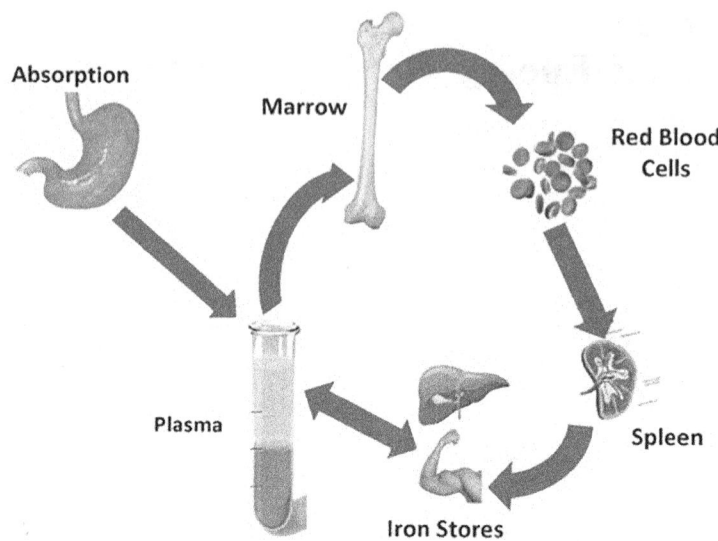

Fig. 10.1 The iron cycle. Iron is absorbed in the stomach and the first portions of the jejunum and transferred to the stores in the liver and muscles through plasma transferrin. At the end of their survival, the red blood cells pass iron to the spleen histiocytes; then iron is transferred (via transferrin) to ferritin in the stores (liver and muscles), from where it is mobilized to the marrow when required

During their childbearing years, women lose about 2.5 mg of iron during each menstrual cycle, which is about the same amount taken in with food. However, women with metrorrhagia (blood loss between periods) and menorrhagia (excessive blood loss during a period) lose between 8 and 15 mg monthly. This means that over 2–4 years, iron stores would become empty, and anemia would develop and get rapidly worse. In males, blood loss is much less frequent.

Another important concept is that iron deficiency is mostly due to blood losses, whilst reduced absorption or dietary deficiency is rare, at least in rich countries where diet is varied and abundant. Other causes affecting iron balance are the very frequent worm infestations, especially Ancylostoma (Hookworm): this worm attaches to the wall of the duodenum, leading to chronic blood losses.

Anemia does not only cause fatigue, but it also reduces the ability to work and study, especially in adolescents. During the first years of adolescent's fertile life ('menarche'), period abnormalities are frequent and need to be identified as early as possible; therefore, maternal supervision is important. Luckily, within a couple of years, periods become regular and acquire the characteristics that they will have in adulthood.

Of relevance, the risk of death during and after delivery increases in young and adult women with anemia, a fact that is not rare in developing countries. Let's not forget that iron is also essential to producing myoglobin. This protein transfers oxygen from hemoglobin to the mitochondria, where there are other iron-containing

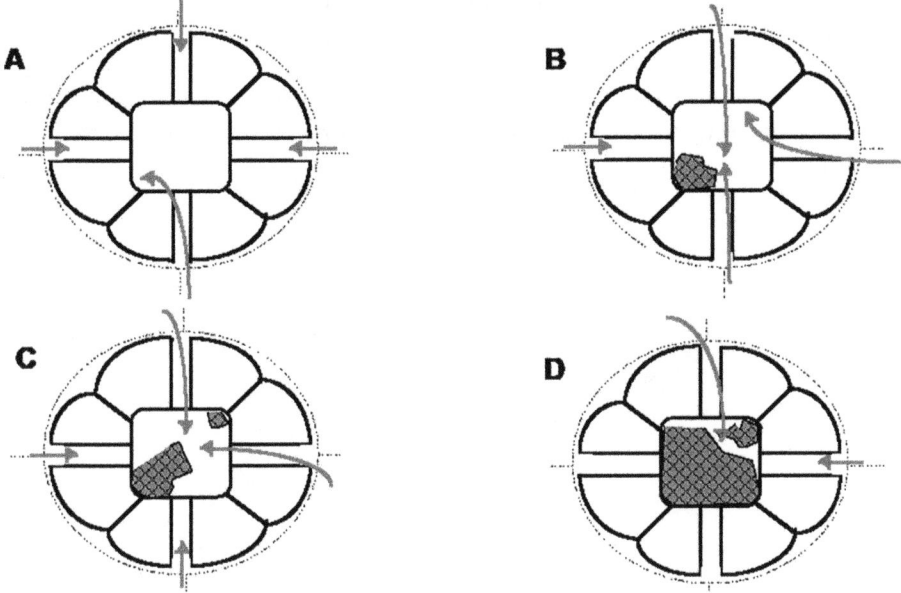

Fig. 10.2 Ferritin: the mechanism of iron storage. (**a–d**) How iron intake (red arrows) occurs through the pores between ferritin molecule subunits (4 highlighted by the red star). Iron is stored in the central area (squared of the sub-units and is shown in blue. (**a**) No iron (unsaturated ferritin). (**d**) Fully saturated ferritin. (**b, c**) Intermediate stages of saturation

proteins, the cytochromes. Thus, if there is a lack of iron, the entire function of the oxygen-transport chain is hampered. Myoglobin is present in the muscles and its reduction may partly explain why we feel tired in the case of iron deficiency. Another important fact is that free iron is toxic to tissues, which is why it is always bound to ferritin in the stores. Importantly, a small amount of iron-saturated ferritin is present in the blood, in balance with the tissue ferritin. Its measurement, therefore, is particularly useful for determining iron reserves.

Anemia can be indolent and thus, diagnosis may be delayed. However, if we consider men and women beyond their fifties, iron deficiency and anemia are most frequently caused by bowel cancer and, so, if iron deficiency is diagnosed early, it can save lives.

To produce blood cells, the body also needs proteins, minerals, and vitamins, in a balanced diet. The vitamins that directly influence blood formation are vitamin B9 (which is folic acid) and vitamin B12. Vitamin B9 is present in vegetables, whereas B12 is only obtainable from the meat of animals. Therefore, vegetarians and vegans are at high risk of becoming anemic in the long run. Vitamin B12 deficiency (previously known as 'pernicious anemia'), was considered a type of leukemia since it often caused death. Differently from most iron deficiencies, the deficiency of vitamins important for hematopoiesis is due to their absence in the diet or abnormal absorption mechanisms. The requirement of vitamin B12 is minimal (about one microgram daily) and the liver contains huge amounts of it. Therefore, this type of anemia develops after years of poor absorption! Before colonization, the American Indians once a year used to eat raw liver from bison which is rich in iron, vitamin B12, and folic acid. Other micronutrients, such as copper and vitamins A, B1, C, and D are important for hematopoiesis and therefore are important elements of our diet.

Chapter 11
When Blood Does Not Clot Properly (Hemophilia)

The Clotting Process

The hemostasis mechanism starts from the platelets, which make the initially deposited plug. To resist blood pressure, there must be sufficient platelets in a clot. If not, blood loss cannot be stopped, or stopped with significant delay. It is thought that the minimum number of platelets necessary to stop a hemorrhage is between 50,000 and 80,000, and when below 10,000 platelets, bleeding can be spontaneous.

Platelet numbers can be lower than normal as the result of an attack by antibodies (especially auto-antibodies) or because megakaryocytes do not produce enough of them. In both of these scenarios, we use the term of 'thrombocytopenia'.

In some cases, platelets can be normal in number but cannot bind to each other because they are not able to release the sticky proteins that join them together or may be unable to activate blood coagulation. When this happens, we talk about 'Platelet Diseases', that can be either hereditary or acquired (in the latter case mostly from drugs).

Hemorrhagic (or Bleeding) disorders (or Bleeds) (due to defects in clotting) have been known for millennia. In the Talmud, (the collection of Rabbinic laws and traditions), there is a scripture that bans circumcision (the cutting of the foreskin, prescribed by the Jewish and the Muslim religions) in a child if two siblings had previously died of hemorrhage after the cut. In the Bible, there is a tale of a woman who bled for many years before touching the edge of Jesus's tunic. Around 1000 AD, an Arabian doctor, Abu Khasim, described families where some members had died from hemorrhages. In 1803, the first study was published with a genealogic tree documenting a familial bleeding disorder encompassing three generations. The author was John Conrad Otto, a doctor from Philadelphia, who described these patients as "hemorrhagic". The term hemophilia was coined by Shönlein, a Professor from the University of Zurich, and his student Hopff. All the other congenital hemorrhagic diseases based on faulty or missing components of the blood clotting

© The Author(s), under exclusive license to Springer Nature Switzerland AG 2025
G. Mariani et al., *Blood: The Science, History, and Mysteries of Life's Vital Flow*, https://doi.org/10.1007/978-3-031-92481-1_11

system were described between 1926 and 1970. The 'coagulation proteins' were called Factors, IXIII. They circulate in the blood and through interaction with platelets, vessel walls, and granulocytes can stop the loss of blood. Hemorrhages can be external if the blood pours out from the body, internal if it occurs within the tissues (brain, muscles) or in the cavities lined with mucous membranes (bowel, respiratory system, and urinary system). The blood loss is stopped by its transformation from a liquid to a solid form, the clot. Proteins participating in blood coagulation are of three types: (i) those that are large and sticky, (ii) those that accelerate the process and (iii) the smaller ones, which are enzymes. The sticky proteins (the scientific name is "adhesive") are fibrinogen and von Willebrand factor, the accelerators are factors V and VIII and all the others are enzymes (Table 6.2 and Fig. 11.1).

The distinction between the various bleeding disorders relates to the fact that each is caused by the loss of activity of a specific protein due to a gene mutation. Only at the end of the last century were these gene defects described in detail and the corresponding deficient factors "cloned" (which means reproduced in the laboratory). But how is this important protective mechanism activated? What occurs is a sort of cascade where enzymes and accelerators are progressively involved till the formation of thrombin which transforms fibrinogen into a net called Fibrin (Fig. 11.1).

If this mechanism fails, a small cut or wound would be enough for an individual to continue to bleed for a long time as is the case of a stomach ulcer. Everything starts from the vessel wall of an artery, a vein, or a capillary: damage to the wall activates the platelets and the sticky proteins together with the clotting factors. The sticky proteins let the platelets adhere to each other and to the damaged endothelial

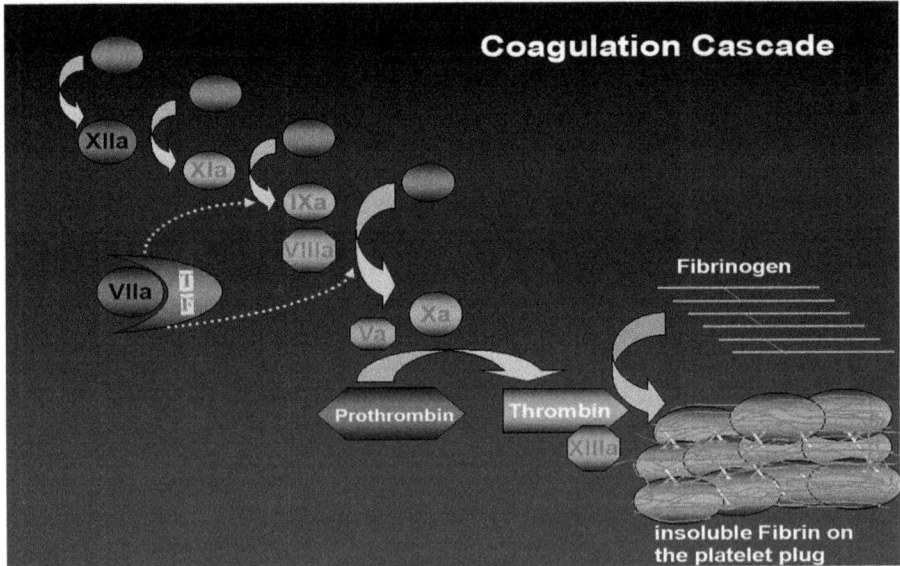

Fig. 11.1 The coagulation cascade

area. The clotting cascade eventually leads to the production of a small, very active enzyme, called thrombin, which cements the platelets to one another and consolidates the clot that becomes waterproof and able to resist blood pressure.

Coagulation factors circulate in two forms: proenzymes and enzymes; the latter are identified by the letter 'a', which means 'activated' (Table 11.1). Coagulation can be started either by Factor (F)XIIa or FVIIa (in red). Once a factor is activated, it activates the factors downstream (this explains the term cascade): FXIIa activates FXI; FXIa activates FIX; FIXa activates FX with the help of FVIII; FXa activates Prothrombin (FII) with the help of FV, leading to the production of Thrombin (FIIa) that transforms the soluble Fibrinogen into a mesh of Fibrin, that is finally stabilized by FXIII.

Almost all hemorrhagic diseases belong to the so-called 'Rare Diseases'. These can affect all populations and every ethnicity around the world, with a well known prevalence. For these disorders, there are specific standards for diagnosis, and treatment. Disorders of Blood Coagulation affect individuals of both sexes, except for hemophilia (there are two types, A and B) In these two hemorrhagic diseases, only males are affected because the genes (those coding for relevant coagulation factors) are located on the X chromosome. As females have two chromosomes (XX), they can compensate for the deficiency through the additional, healthy chromosome X, while males with only one chromosome X (XY), cannot do so. Females are referred to as "carriers," and they do not manifest the typical symptoms of the disease.

For example (Fig. 11.2), the Empress Alexandra of Russia, the mother of Alexis, was a hemophilia carrier (XX), and Alexis was affected (XY) was affected by hemophilia, while some of Alexis's sisters were carriers (we do not know which ones). Had they survived, they could have transmitted the disease to their offspring. The Tzar Nicholas II, having passed on his Y chromosome, which does not contain the gene for either of the two coagulation factors, could not help to correct the genetic defect of his son Alexis.

Not all hemorrhagic diseases have the same symptoms: hemophilias are characterized by hemorrhages into the joints (especially in the knees, ankles, and elbows), whilst other disorders manifest themselves mainly with hemorrhages in mucous membranes* or the skin. Moreover, not all individuals affected by hemophilia have the same disease severity. Some have mild symptoms (bruises) whilst others suffer from life-threatening hemorrhages (cerebral or bleeds in the gastrointestinal tract).

Sometimes, the genetic transmission of a bleeding disorder may not be as clear as that shown in Fig. 11.2. This can be due to the lack of male descendants in one or more generations or to mild bleeding manifestations that passed unobserved. However, recent molecular genetic analysis has indicated that in up to 50% of hemophilia cases, mutations are spontaneous and, therefore are considered as de novo (out of the blue) mutations.

The hemostasis mechanism starts from the platelets, that create the initially deposited plug. To resist blood pressure, there must be a sufficient number of effective platelets in the clot. If not, blood loss cannot be stopped or stopped with significant delay. It is postulated that the minimum number of platelets necessary to stop

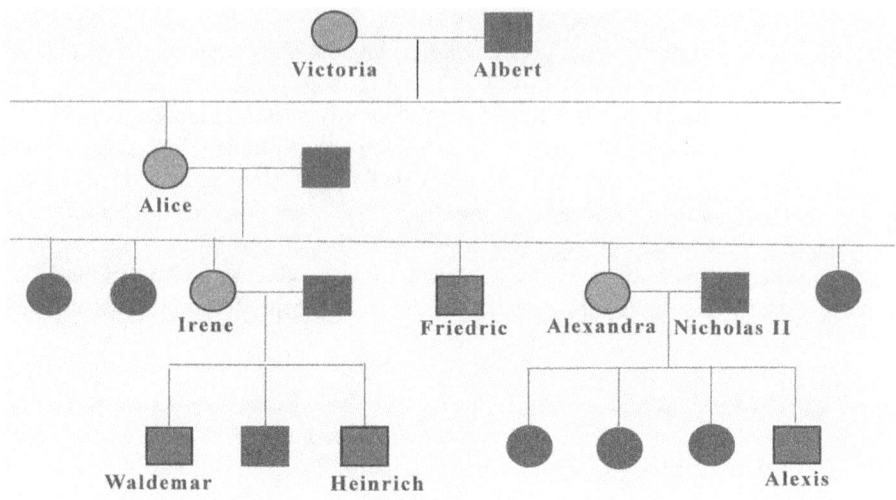

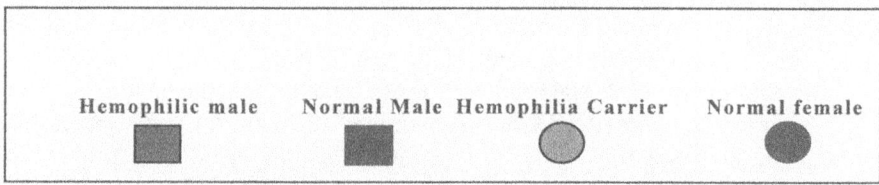

Fig. 11.2 Hemophilia inheritance as shown by the Victoria Queen of the United Kingdom and Ireland family tree

a hemorrhage is between 50,000 and 80,000, and when below 10,000 platelets, bleeding can be spontaneous.

Platelet numbers can be lower than normal as the result of an attack by antibodies (especially auto-antibodies) or because megakaryocytes do not produce enough of them. In both scenarios, we talk about thrombocytopenia.

In some cases, platelets can be normal in number but cannot bind to each other because they are not able to release the sticky proteins that are necessary join them together or lack of the proteins able to activate blood coagulation. When this happens, we talk about thrombocytopathy, which can be either hereditary or acquired (in this case mostly from drugs).

Until now, we have talked about hereditary hemorrhagic disorders, but there are also frequent acquired bleeding disorders. In general, these are systemic and secondary to a liver diseases. An enlarged spleen can worsen bleeding by trapping more platelets.

Chapter 12
When There Is Too Much Clotting (Thrombosis)

Thrombosis is a clinical event caused by the formation of a clot inside a vessel. The thrombus is composed of platelets, red blood cells, and fibrin in various proportions, and it can totally or partially obstruct a blood vessel (vein, artery, capillary). The thrombus composition depends on the site where it forms: in the veins, it is redder because it contains many red blood cells, while in the arteries, it is whiter because platelets are more represented.

It is a fact that thrombosis, be it arterial, venous, or in small vessels, is a leading cause of death throughout the world.

In the case of venous thrombosis, blood accumulates in the upstream limbs and tissues, which become engorged, and 'edema' (*swelling caused by excess extra-vascular fluids*) ensues. If the thrombus is fragile, part of it can break away from the vessel wall and be propelled toward the lung. Depending on the size of this piece of thrombus (called 'embolus'), it may obstruct a small or a major vessel of the lung, the first filter organ that it finds. This phenomenon is called 'thrombo-embolism'.

Years ago, journalists all over the world wrote articles about 'killer flights' (those between London and Sydney) because of the occurrence of several episodes of thromboembolism that were seen after these long plane journeys. This was not related to the boredom of passengers staying seated with their legs curled up and watching film repeats for 20 hours, but to episodes that occurred after their arrival: some travelers walking into the terminal developed severe and sudden respiratory difficulties. Some of the passengers, despite being immediately seen by emergency medics at the airport, died within a few hours in the local hospital. As a result of this, the Australian Thrombosis and Hemostasis Society undertook a study and concluded that these were episodes of fatal thrombo-embolism, rare but dramatic events (occurring in 1 out of 2 million travelers). However, this study also indicates that if there are other risk factors such as obesity, advanced age, smoking or previous episodes of thromboembolism, the frequency of the event may be 20 times higher!

The same fate (death following pulmonary embolism) hit a famous war correspondent of NBC (the largest American television network), David Bloom, who

G. Mariani et al., *Blood: The Science, History, and Mysteries of Life's Vital Flow*, https://doi.org/10.1007/978-3-031-92481-1_12

followed American troops on war operations in Iraq. Sitting in an uncomfortable armored vehicle that moved through the deserts and dirt roads, he was broadcasting, live, the fighting. Just before the accident, Bloom called his wife on a satellite telephone and told her that he felt an odd discomfort in his legs. Because of this, he asked the driver to stop the vehicle, and he jumped off to stretch his legs with a high risk of being killed. After a short walk, he collapsed to the ground with severe breathing difficulties: he was killed, not by a bullet, but from an embolus mobilized by his legs!

However, the standard risk factors (obesity, diabetes, sedentary behavior, advanced age, hypertension) cannot explain these events in young people in their twenties, thirties, or forties. Interestingly, cases of thrombosis have occurred in celebrities, including athletes such as the tennis player Serena Williams and the Abbagnale brothers who won five Olympic gold medals for canoeing, and fortunately, not all thromboses and pulmonary embolisms are fatal.

In the case of arterial thrombosis, the organ downstream will receive less blood, an event we call 'ischemia' (from Greek isch = reduction and aemia = blood) or an 'infarct' (from Latin infarctus = trapped inside) since blood cannot be pushed forward due to the lack of circulation.

In the arteries, the mechanism that leads to the formation of a thrombus occurs only if the vessel wall is damaged due to the presence of atherosclerotic plaques (atherothrombosis). These plaques are the consequence of a damage caused to the vessel by high levels of cholesterol and hypertension.

Since an arterial thrombus is rich in platelets, effective drugs are those that inhibit the ability of platelets to aggregate. Aspirin and antiplatelet agents are efficient, especially in preventing recurrences (secondary prevention) of a myocardial infarct or a cerebral stroke. Aspirin contains an ingredient that has been known for more than 100 years, Acetylsalicylic acid, which was originally extracted from the weeping willow trees. However, other more efficacious antiplatelet agents are available and are used alone or in association with aspirin. The balance between hemorrhage and the prevention of thrombosis (called 'risk/benefit ratio') is very favorable as the main side effect, hemorrhage, is rare. Another advantage is that these drugs do not require laboratory monitoring.

In the veins, the main mechanism leading to thrombus formation is the reduction of blood flow velocity (Chap. 9) which favors an increase in blood coagulability. This explains why in the prevention and treatment of venous thrombosis and thrombo-embolism, anticoagulants are the treatment of choice. The most used anticoagulants are those that interfere with the synthesis of those coagulation factors that are dependent on vitamin K metabolism (factor II, VII, IX, and X). Even though these are old drugs, millions of people are still using them. The clinical presentation of venous thrombosis is related to the formation of a thrombus, especially in the leg veins, very rarely in other organs (i.e. the brain and the intestine). A thrombus obstructing a leg vein originates inside a vein valve, increases in size, and eventually causes a complete obstruction of the vessel. Upstream, in the ankles, the venules become engorged with blood, leading to limb swelling.

If treatment is not initiated, a downstream part of the thrombus can break away and reach a distant organ: this is the mechanism of embolism, which, in the case of the limb veins, affects the lung (pulmonary embolism) and if the embolus is large, can cause a 'sudden death'. But one wonders, how does the clot find the energy to move, since the blood flow is blocked? Do you remember the fatal death after the killer flights? During a flight, the venous circulation is slowed down due to physical inactivity, but when the traveler is standing and walks the leg muscles compress the veins, and the thrombus is propelled upwards. Another important element to consider in these cases is dehydration: on a plane and in the desert (as in the case of Bloom), the air is very dry and the blood becomes more 'dense'.

Anticoagulants are the most effective drugs in preventing lung embolisms and the formation of a thrombus in the heart during atrial fibrillation. In this case, the embolus is not propelled towards the lung but towards the arteries of the brain. The oldest and most established anticoagulants are heparin (given systemically, intravenously or subcutaneously) and coumarin derivatives like warfarin and acenocoumarol, for oral use. These anticoagulants are still widely used in clinical practice, but they have the disadvantage of requiring frequent laboratory testing for monitoring. As alternatives to coumarin derivatives, new anticoagulants (dabigatran, rivaroxaban, apixaban, edoxaban, and others being developed) are now used, because they do not require laboratory monitoring and bear a lower hemorrhagic risk.

Globally, it is a fact that 1 in 4 individuals die from the consequences of a thrombosis. The most frequent clinical presentation is myocardial infarction, followed by cerebral stroke (thrombosis or hemorrhage) and venous thromboembolism. The dramatic extent of the morbidity and mortality caused by thrombosis requires approaches based on primary prevention; secondary prevention measures are also important, to avoid recurrences. The consensus is that the most efficient mechanisms of prevention (either primary or secondary) are healthy lifestyles: avoiding smoking, keeping an optimal body weight, doing regular physical activity, limiting animal fats in the diet, avoiding hypercaloric foods, alcohol, and increasing the consumption of fruits and vegetables.

The risk of travel-related thrombosis may have been over-emphasized because it is a very rare event occurring after flights over large distances. To reduce this risk, walking in the aisles and simple leg exercises are recommended, together with drinking plenty of water and avoiding excessive food and alcohol intake.

Generally, it is thought that thrombosis prevention is based on laboratory tests providing information about the individual's risk. In arterial thrombosis, the best-known risk factor is the increase in blood cholesterol, especially of LDL (low-density lipoproteins; the so-called 'bad cholesterol'). This blood test is only a generic indicator, useful to suggest lifestyle changes, and it does not obligatory require the need to take drugs that lower cholesterol such as statins. Likewise, there are no laboratory tests that can accurately predict the risk of developing infarcts and stroke.

Regarding venous thrombosis, there are a few genetic mutations that favor the production of thrombin through a 'gain of function' mechanism (see Chap. 11), which mostly represents a risk factor for venous thrombosis.

These mutations were found positive with a higher prevalence in the victims of killer flights; Bloom, also, was positive. However, these are risk factors that alone do not cause thrombosis and the consensus is that anti-thrombotic management in carriers of these mutations should not be prescribed unless other risk factors are present, considering that there is also the risk of labeling ill individuals with a genetic variation a fact that can have psychological implications.

From a scientific point of view, it is ridiculous and uneconomical to perform genetic tests that are part of pre-packaged panels, because they represent a risk of uncertain significance for venous and arterial thrombosis. Instead, it is more important to stress that personal, clinical, and family histories are the most powerful tools for identifying a thrombotic risk. Concerning this issue, other important aspects to evaluate are physical inactivity, obesity, and the so-called 'metabolic syndrome', important determinants of thrombosis that require a lifestyle change. In fact, in the metabolic Syndrome, the metabolism slows down, with an accumulation of non-metabolized fats stored in any site of the body. Is it possible to stop or reverse this process? Firstly, lifestyle must be corrected: this involves giving up smoking, increasing physical exercise, and reducing obesity as well as alcohol intake. Only in the next stage should the syndrome be treated with drugs. In fact, without the correction of lifestyle, there is little chance of success.

Since thrombosis can occur in many different organs, the symptoms depend on the organ affected and management requires a multidisciplinary approach.

Finally, there is another catastrophic type of thrombosis the one occurring in the small vessels, such as arterioles and capillaries. What is unusual is that symptoms involve many organs and systems and are both thrombotic and hemorrhagic. The most evident symptoms are cutaneous hemorrhages, ecchymosis, petechiae, hematomas, and skin necrosis*, but what occurs in the skin capillaries also takes place in other organs and tissues. In this type of thrombosis, there is a mixed mechanism involving, both thrombin and platelets. Red blood cells are also involved since they are destroyed by the microthrombi that form in the capillaries with subsequent release of hemoglobin into the bloodstream. This phenomenon is called 'micro-angiopathic anemia' and takes place in a group of diseases including DIC (disseminated intravascular coagulation) and Thrombotic Thrombocytopenic Purpura (TTP) and is associated with a high rate of mortality. These diseases are also denominated 'thrombo-hemorrhagic' disorders since hemorrhages and thromboses occur simultaneously.

Part IV
Blood and Disease Management

Chapter 13
Transfusion of Blood and Blood Components

History of First Transfusions

Transfusion is based on the injection of blood or one of its fractions into the circulation of a recipient. In the case of plasma, or plasma-derived products, the term currently used is 'infusion'. The AIDS and hepatitis dramas have rendered transfusion a safe practice by the introduction of physical and chemical methods effective to kill blood-borne microorganisms.

The first transfusion was given to Naaman, a Syrian General: his 'sick' blood was taken and replaced with new blood, a kind of exchange-transfusion* that, according to the narrative, had healed him from leprosy. In the Odyssey, to resuscitate the fortune teller Tiresia, Ulysses transfused her with the blood of two sheep given as a present from the sorceress Circe. Galenus anticipated the concept of 'transfusion' as the possibility of removing corrupted blood from the body and replacing it with transfused healthy blood.

However, we have to wait till 1664, when the first blood transfusions were carried out between dogs for scientific purposes. Transfusions amongst other species followed.

At the beginning of the nineteenth century, doctors again showed interest in transfusion, considering the severe and often fatal hemorrhages that occurred during or after child delivery. In this desperate situation, direct transfusions from one arm to the other were often tried. However, even if the equipment improved, the results were not at all reassuring. In 1873, a Polish doctor, Franz Gasellius, carried out research on blood transfusion by analyzing clinical notes, records, and publications related to its previous use. The results of the analysis were disconcerting: mortality attributable to blood transfusion was 56%, a percentage similar to that obtained by Dr. James Blundell (50%) who at the beginning of 1800 transfused 10 patients of whom 5 passed away. In 1818, Blundell was the first to perform a direct transfusion from one arm to another, and even considering the high mortality, the results did not appear to discourage him. This was because of the extremely high mortality of post-partum hemorrhages, which at that time were close to 100%. These studies provided the basis of a new method that turned out to be very useful: the birth of Medical Statistics. In 1840 a French Doctor, Pierre-Charles Alexandre Louis started to collect data from patients using standard questionnaires, taking accurate notes of the answers, and comparing the data with treatment outcomes. The data acquired from his numerous patients were presented at meetings organized by scientific societies (including the English Royal Medical Society and Royal College of Physicians in London), but the medical community continued to consider blood transfusion a dangerous practice and, therefore was abandoned again.

So, successful blood transfusion is a relatively recent achievement. But why has this simple procedure required so much time to develop? There were several unsolved problems;

- Blood clots when outside the body
- Blood has a relatively short shelf-life
- It can transmit pathogens
- There is a variable degree of incompatibility between individuals

The problem of clotting was solved by adding an anticoagulant, tri-sodium-citrate to blood: the first transfusion with anticoagulated blood was carried out in 1914 by Hustin, a Belgian. His studies and those of others demonstrated that sodium citrate was a safe and efficient anticoagulant. This substance binds the calcium in the blood, an element essential for its coagulation.

In addition, a serious issue is the transfer of blood and plasma between countries (globalization): blood can be obtained in developing countries from poorly paid donors and industrially processed in the USA or Europe where it gains a great deal of value.

The problem of contamination with pathogens is a serious issue; when exposed to the environment, it can be a kind of growth medium for bacteria, fungi, and viruses. With globalization, a particular risk came to light, since different pathogens can be present in the blood of populations living in distant and distinct areas of the world. Perishability is another aspect that, for many years, has prevented blood from being exported: blood cells deteriorate in a relatively short time, and its storage in fridges only delays this by a few hours.

But let us proceed in sequence: Why and how were blood transfusion and fractionation introduced?

How It All Started

Everything started during the Spanish Civil War. The wounded ran the risk of dying because of bleeding. A Canadian surgeon, Norman Bethune (Fig. 13.1), a volunteer in the Republican army, had the idea of organizing a frontline transfusion system. Norman was convinced that blood transfusions would have saved many lives.

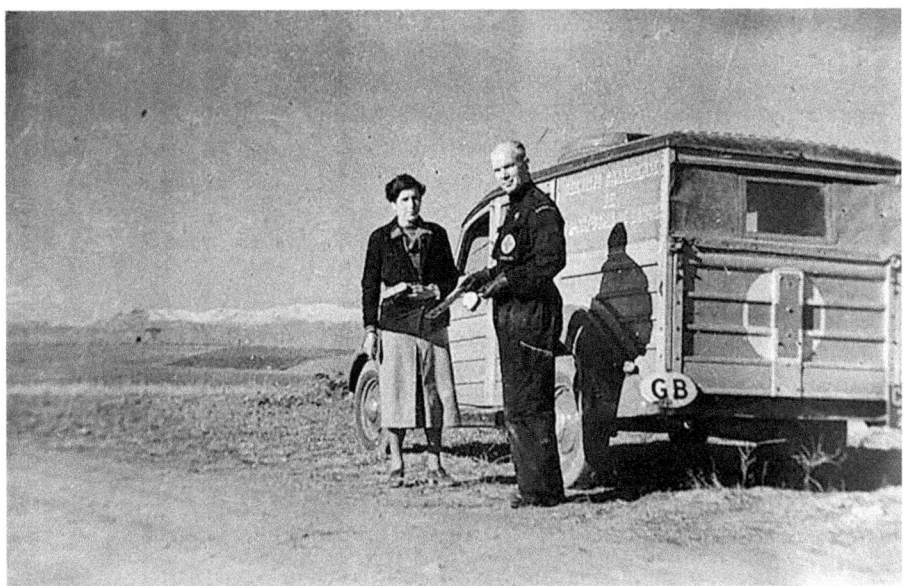

Fig. 13.1 A rare image of Norman Bethune with his mobile blood bank in Spain during the Civil War

Hence, he organized a very basic mobile blood bank using clean sterilized bottles of milk or wine to collect blood that was kept in a liquid state with a salt i.e. sodium citrate. Blood taken from volunteers was stored in fridges for up to one week: when needed on the battlefield, Bethune arrived with his lorry containing a portable fridge (packed with ice cubes). He carried out blood group identification by taking a sample from a finger and hence transfused compatible blood. This heroic organization proved that stored blood could work and was used for many months on the battlefields. When in Madrid, he met a Spanish hematologist, Federico Duran Jorda, who understood the importance of Bethune's idea and organized a safer and more scientific transfusion center in Barcelona. There, Federico opened a center that was advanced for those times: blood was collected in sterilized bottles containing citrate, oxygenated with filtered air, and transfused using a system of rubber tubes he had designed. The most important innovation was the fact that he transfused only blood group O, the universal donor blood group. Moreover, he observed that the time of blood storage could be prolonged for up to two weeks. This approach simplified and expedited much of the transfusion procedures so that the Centro de Transfusion de Sangre Barcelona at the end of the 1930s managed to withdraw blood from 75 donors per hour. Another innovation was that blood was screened for syphilis, and its safety was checked using a questionnaire focused on the donor's health state. When Francisco Franco conquered Barcelona, Federico Duran Jorda fled to London, where his innovative ideas were appreciated. Duran Jorda's practical idea of using only the blood of group O as a universal donor represented a great simplification of the procedure.

In 1938–1939, prior to the second world war, the preparations to defend London were well underway: it was commonly believed that the Luftwaffe would bomb the city every day from the start of the war. Federico Duran Jorda met Janet Vaughan, who graduated in Medicine in Oxford and had acquired a grant from the Rockefeller Institute in New York. Janet was brilliant, but as a woman she had significant difficulties at the beginning of her career. However, Virginia Woolf (the known writer and women's rights activist was her cousin) educated her to fight her corner. As a hematologist, she realized that it was necessary to organize a transfusion service based on the storage of blood. However, it would have been impossible to recruit voluntary donors during the bombing and to arrange a system based on direct arm-to-arm donations. Hence, Janet and Federico, supported by the Medical Research Council (MRC), proposed a network of four transfusion centers in peripheral and strategic sites in London. To store blood, milk bottles were chosen which were soon renamed Vaughan's bottles. In the first year of the war, there was no bombing, thus the centers were not activated. Janet and her colleagues identified 8000 potential donors having blood group "O".

One day, on the first of September 1939, she received a telegram from the MRC instructing her to start taking blood. Initially, blood was used for the injured at Dunkerque. But by the 7th of September 1940, a sunny day brought a wave of German bombers over the city. The blood transfusion system worked very well: a few minutes before the beginning of the bombing, the alarm was sent from Dover to the hospitals in the areas under attack; hospitals alerted their transfusion center of reference and blood arrived before the injured persons reached the emergency rooms. Car drivers were real heroes during these events: they drove regardless of the bombs dropping around them and even during the nights with no lights on since they knew their areas very well. The system worked admirably for the entire duration of the war. Strangely, there are no statistics available, but the Units of blood that Janet withdrew amounted to about 70,000 gallons (imperial gallon = 4.5 liters). If we consider that one unit of blood consists of 450 ml, 700,000 units of blood group O were taken during the war in London. Fortunately, this blood group is present in 44% of the UK population. The media reported that during that time, from 10 to 30% of the injured required blood transfusions. Other cities in the UK adopted the system of Janet Vaughan and Duran Jorda.

Transfusion of Blood Products

On the other side of the Atlantic, the approach was different from the beginning: the consensus was that for those injured or severely traumatized, blood fractions capable of restoring blood volume had to be the first-choice therapy. Therefore, research was focused on plasma and plasma fractions, especially albumin. As we have seen, plasma represents little more than 50% of the blood volume and contains an array of proteins, some in large quantities and a few very rare. The idea that plasma and plasma-derived products could solve the problem of shock in injured people was based on observations made during the First World War. So, Dr. Charles Drew pursued this strategy.

Charles was an African American doctor who became famous for his graduation degree paper entitled Blood Bank, a new concept for those times. With a few colleagues, he opened a laboratory in the New York Presbyterian Hospital to study blood and plasma storage. Since the war in Europe had already started, he was summoned to Harvard University in Boston to organize the transfusion support program 'Plasma for Britain'. Plasma has many advantages over whole blood (is handy, transportable, and freezable) but could be contaminated with microorganisms during separation, and the British called it 'liquid dynamite'. Drew prepared well-defined methods for the withdrawal and separation of blood, isolating it from air contaminants and setting up a screening for known blood-borne infections, syphilis, and malaria. The project was highly appreciated by the public and long donor queues formed outside the hospitals. Around 15,000 vials of plasma were produced, and Drew became an international hero. However, the executives of the Red Cross decided that vials from Blacks should be identified with a label, so Drew resigned and returned to teach at the African-American Howard University in Washington. However, this racial issue did not stop there, it took decades before the Red Cross accepted that there was no difference between black blood and white blood.

In the USA, with the approach of war, the government recruited an internationally famous protein chemist, Edwin J. Cohn. The idea was already there: plasma and albumin could solve the problems in injured people with massive trauma and severe burns. Cohn hypothesized that by infusing anti-shock proteins—the proteins that attract water from the tissues—blood volume would be restored. In this way, there were no risks of contamination, infections, or blood instability. Cohn was a determined scientist and an authority in the field. He managed to create the National Research Defense Committee and a department for Scientific Research and Development. He involved numerous American Universities and contracted out the research he could not do himself. Moreover, for large-scale experiments, he involved industries whose technical experts were trained by his research group. Nobody could deny support to him as he had a government role in coordinating this strategic activity.

A transfusion committee was established to determine which of the two approaches, plasma or whole blood, would have been the most appropriate. Finally, Cohn was given the green light for plasma fractionation, and within one year, he proposed a practical method of plasma separation into 5 fractions, from I to V. The announcement of these scientific results was made in 1940, but later, nothing was made known to the public and the project became a secret of the State, like the Manhattan Project (the atomic bomb).

Fraction V had the advantage of being stable even at room temperature, containing almost exclusively albumin and therefore with a strong oncotic power. After the safety experiments performed in healthy volunteers, all the available albumin was sent to Pearl Harbor by request of the Navy, where the Japanese attack had already occurred. The albumin was successfully used for a few critically ill sailors, especially those with severe burns. Unfortunately, the albumin arrived 4 days after the attack, had it arrived earlier, more lives could have been saved.

So, Cohn developed two plasma products to use for war injuries: whole plasma in powder form (obtained by a procedure called 'Lyophilization'*) and purified albumin, both easily transportable and stable for a reasonable time at room temperature. Cohn moved laboratory bench fractionation to an industrial scale: he used big steel containers, where thousands of liters of plasma sourced from multiple donations were processed. Since 3.6 blood donations were required to produce one unit of albumin, the concept of a plasma pool (a large amount resulting from the mixing of plasma sourced from up to a thousand donors) became an important step for large-scale production. Cohn's method was progressively refined and when he believed it to be fully developed, it was taught to staffs sent from nine pharmaceutical companies that became responsible for the production on a national scale.

A national campaign was organized by the Red Cross to encourage donations: large financial and workers' organizations led periodic campaigns to implement the program. Unsurprisingly, two-thirds of the donors were women, as most of the young male adults were fighting at the frontline!

Cohn did not stop there, he maintained supervision of the industrial production of albumin for a long period. But he was a chemist, not a doctor. The frontline surgeons soon realized that albumin and lyophilized plasma were useful to restore the blood volume but could not solve the problem of hypoxia, that is, the reduced oxygen supply to the tissues due to the loss of hemoglobin. Hypoxia is one of the most important causes of traumatic shock, a complex phenomenon which is the final step of a series of events culminating in widespread tissue damage. In short, capillaries and arterioles initially undergo vasoconstriction to adapt to the reduction in blood volume, and subsequently vessel paralysis occurs, followed by shock (drop in blood pressure). This disaster is initiated by capillary paralysis caused by hypoxia and the release of inflammatory substances. Albumin can temporarily restore the blood volume but not the lack of oxygen.

On this basis, the American army surgeons started requiring units of whole blood, but Washington replied in a bureaucratic way, saying that the decision had been made that it would not be possible to organize the transfer of large quantities of blood to the frontline operating theatres. The problem was not solved but a surgeon, Edward Churchill who was opreating on the front line, started to bombard Washington with requests for blood. On the other side of the ocean, the Surgeon General (the Minister of Health in the USA) was an orthopedic surgeon who was reluctant to change the status quo. Thus, Churchill decided to do everything independently and at the risk of a court-martial, asked the industry directly for all he needed: bottles, tubes, and needles. He started to collect blood during the invasion of Italy. A journalist from the New York Times became aware of this story and wrote an article entitled 'Fresh Blood Saves Soldiers' lives in Sicily, while plasma appears to be inadequate'.

In England, Paul Hawley (a surgeon responsible for the Northern European war theatre, was awaiting the landings in Normandy and tried to set up a way of using whole blood, but again the Surgeon General refused. So, Hawley created a team to organize donations in England since at that time, there were one and a half million American Soldiers stationed there. However, considering that within 6 months most soldiers had to fight, the number of potential donors would have been reduced dramatically. In addition, another serious problem occurred: the equipment required for the transfusions was stuck in the harbor in New York, lost amidst huge quantities of materials to be sent for the war effort. So, Hawley stocked up vans with standard bottles used locally and started to organize donations. On the first day of the Normandy landing, the number of casualties was enormous, and it quickly became clear that available donations would not be sufficient. Hawley's group realized that with a war front extending hundreds of kilometers and the forthcoming invasion of Germany, a colossal amount of blood would be necessary. Therefore, they made a final desperate request to Washington. The answer was: The Surgeon General has expressed the opinion that if the Hawley Centre needs blood, then it should have it. Finally, the old bureaucrat conceded! Blood supplies started to arrive when the Allied forces entered Paris.

But there was also the Pacific front to consider, which seemed never ending with the most terrible theatres of death being those of IwoJima and Okinawa. Therefore, the Red Cross, following the request of the Surgeon General organized a campaign for blood collection of group O to be sent to the frontlines along with lyophilized plasma and albumin. Finally, blood arrived on the beaches of the Pacific islands during the battles and several historical photos show stretchers on the shore with injured soldiers being transfused with blood, plasma, or albumin while waiting to be transferred to hospital ships. Hence, the battle between bureaucracy and frontline American doctors ended without any winners or losers!

The Birth of Transfusion Programs Worldwide

After World War II, transfusion programs started to function everywhere in Europe. The American research and the war experience created the basis for future transfusion organizations as well as blood fractionation, which became an industrial activity of great economic success.

In the beginning, there was a poorly coordinated development of blood banks. In 1952, transfusion in France became regulated by a specific law. This law created a network of blood banks within the Public Health Program and transferred any transfusion activity to this organization. Additionally, the law regulated the participation of industries in the production of blood derivatives and fractions. The law highlighted the concept that blood donation was a voluntary act having an important social impact. Soon afterward, all the other Western European countries developed coordinated transfusion systems. In Poland, the only country in the Soviet block, blood donation remained voluntary under the coordination of the Red Cross. This was due to the great Ludwig Hirszferlds (see later), who miraculously escaped the massacre of the Warsaw ghetto and became the heart and soul of the organization.

In Japan, blood transfusion became of extreme importance for public health following the dropping of atomic bombs on Hiroshima and Nagasaki. As a consequence, after the Armistice (August 1945), the USA sent Colonel Murray Sanders, an American microbiologist, to investigate the public health situation and look for the laboratories where the intelligence service had reported that bacteriological weapons had been prepared. To tell the truth, this was the primary purpose of his visit. Once off the ship, Sanders unexpectedly found Ryoichy Naito waiting for him. According to the USA intelligence, Naito was believed to be the head of the development program for bacteriological weapons. Naito had a photo of Sanders and warmly welcomed him. Naito had been working together with others who were later identified as war criminals responsible for preparing bacteria and lyophilized toxins, which had been tested out in Manchuria on civilians or prisoners of war. Naito, when cornered, admitted his guilt in a long document but obtained impunity for himself and his collaborators by expressing his willingness to unconditional cooperation. Before the war, Naito had spent six months in the USA (sent by the army on an espionage mission) and bought a lyophilizer from the pharmaceutical company Merck Sharp & Dohme, which he managed to take back to Japan. Once there, he organized a factory to lyophilize plasma, which was destroyed in the last years of the war. However, he had acquired knowledge of a technology that would become very useful to him after the war. When he finished his job of informing the Americans, Naito retired to work as a general practitioner in a small town where he converted to Catholicism. But he soon returned to his previous experiences, considering the economic potential of blood fractionation. He knew that despite the advances in fractionation based on Cohn's work, there was still a big unsolved issue: the treatment of hemophilia.

Factor VIII (the missing protein in hemophilia A (Chap. 10) is a rare plasma protein that is rapidly destroyed at room temperature. It is present in Cohn fraction I, but the quantities are so small that it cannot be used in therapy. To start with, this problem was solved through the cryoprecipitation of plasma factor VIII. The method was relatively simple, could be performed in any transfusion center, and most importantly, allowed hemophiliacs to be treated, though with some difficulty.

The use of cryoprecipitates at the end of the 1960s was the milestone that allowed Europe and the USA to begin modern hemophilia treatment. However, cryoprecipitates had practical and efficacy limitations in that they needed to be stored in freezers and required the admission of hemophilic individuals into hospitals or specialized clinics for treatment.

A fundamental step forward was taken at the beginning of the 1970s when a few pharmaceutical companies began to produce plasma concentrates containing factor VIII (or IX), in the form of lyophilized powders. These concentrates could be stored in a home fridge and reconstituted in small amounts of solvent (hence the term 'concentrates'), that could be injected intravenously in one shot. This important progress provided a significant benefit to individuals with hemophilia. Not only could the patients be treated in specialized clinics, but they also could treat themselves at home. Hemophiliacs learned how to prepare the concentrate and how to inject it intravenously when bleeding occurred or to prevent bleeds by administering concentrates on alternate days.

In 1964, George Hudson realized the importance of blood fractionation while visiting the National Cancer Institute in the USA where his son had been admitted with leukemia. He worked as an engineer for the IBM company and obtained funding from the National Institutes of Health to build one of the first cell separators which was announced in 1965. It was the first automatic system designed to separate cells and plasma from one arm of a donor and to return what was not required to the other arm. The system was further refined and later specific machines for plasma apheresis (plasmapheresis), platelet apheresis (plateletpheresis), and other functions were developed.

It was perhaps with one of these machines that Cohn, a notoriously enthusiastic individual, carried out a demonstration to an audience of scientists. While connected to a machine, he continued explaining how that instrument of wonder was working. At some point during the presentation, the pressure inside the machine increased and the machine exploded—flooding the speaker and those on the closest seats with Cohn's plasma! A connecting tube had become obstructed! But Cohn, not worried at all, detached himself from the machine, cleaned his suit, and continued to talk like nothing had happened.

Today, using cell separators, it is possible to collect the stem cells, a relatively simple procedure that is carried out in blood banks.

Considering the serious problems related to the transmission of hepatitis and HIV infections, the FDA* and EMA* decided to regulate the production of plasma fractions whenever possible using plasma of national origin. In the worst-case scenario, plasma from other countries had to be traceable to the donor. The only exception to this strategy was the United Kingdom, where fractionation of plasma of national origin was banned until 2021 because of the Mad Cow Disease.

Over the years, the availability of locally produced plasma fractions in most European countries has become almost optimal.

In the 1970s, the pharma industry realized that blood fractionation was a golden goose! So, the industry developed plasma fractionation using high technology driven methods that could not be carried out in Transfusion Centers.

Since plasmapheresis required a few hours to be carried out, plasma donors could no longer be voluntary, and so the gap between industry and blood banks became wider, considering the requirement of financial compensation for the donors. Another difference regards the interval needed between donations: voluntary blood donors cannot donate again until after 3 months, whereas paid plasma donors can donate at fortnight intervals because plasma proteins are rapidly replaced.

The main discoveries that led to the practice of blood transfusion and its fractionation are shown in Table 13.1.

Table 13.1 Essential discoveries for the development of blood transfusion and fractionation

Scientist	Idea/hypothesis/ description	Site/date	Details	Blood group	Shelf- life
Karl Landsteiner	Blood groups	Vienna, 1900	Described ABO system and with Wiener (1937) identified the Rh system	Any	–
Richard Luwishon	Anticoagulation for whole blood	New York, 1915	0.2% sodium citrate delays coagulation	Any	1 h
Norman Bethune	Blood transfusion system on the battle field	Spanish Civil War, 1936–39	Whole Blood collected in milk or wine bottles in 3.8% sodium citrate	Compatible blood	1 week
Federico Duran-Jorda	Blood transfusion center	Spanish Civil War, 1936–39	Whole blood collected in standard bottles, oxygenated and 3.8% sodium citrate	O-neg	2 weeks
Janet Vaughan	Blood transfusion center network	London II World War, 1939–1944	Same as above	O-neg	2 weeks
Charles Drew	Concept of blood banking	New York, 1939	Blood storage Separation of plasma	Any	Frozen, Long-lasting
Edwin J Cohn	Plasma fractionation procedures Lyophilization*	USA, World War 2	Plasma fractions I–V	Any	Freeze-drying, Long-lasting
William Murphy	Plastic bags for blood preservation	Korean War, 1950–1953	Plastic bags for blood preservation and separation	Any	4 weeks
Judith Pool	Factor VIII isolation	Palo Alto, California, 1965	Cryo-precipitation	Any	Frozen, Long-lasting
George Judson	Cell separation	NCI Bethesda, 1965	First IBM Cell Separator	Any	For rapid use of blood components

Chapter 14
The Discovery of Blood Groups: The Requirement of Compatible Blood

To make blood transfusion a widely used procedure, a question had to be answered: why did mixing the blood from different individuals could result in red cell aggregation? This issue was solved by an Austrian pathologist, Karl Landsteiner, who in 1900 noticed that the red cell aggregates were different from clots. Moreover, he was convinced that the phenomenon was not due to any blood disease since the samples he analyzed were taken from himself and his coworkers. He recorded the findings obtained by mixing blood samples from different individuals. He noticed a consistent behavior for each individual: the most frequent pattern was called A, the least frequent was called B, and the absence of aggregates was called C. He repeated these experiments by mixing the red blood cells with plasma from different individuals and observed a similar pattern. Later on, he changed the name to the group 'without aggregates', calling it 0 (zero). His data were published in the journal of the Royal and Imperial Society of Clinical Sciences in Vienna (Wiener Klinische Wochenschrift) on the 14th of November 1901. Amongst his conclusions, the one that interested him most was: can our observations help explain the various consequences related to blood transfusion given for therapeutic purposes? This was a conclusion not very much highlighted in his paper. At any rate, his work was awarded the Nobel Prize in 1930. Two years after publication, a fourth blood type, group AB, was discovered (the rarest of the blood groups). This was the Vienna of Freud, Mahler, Klimt, Kokoscka, von Kraft-Ebing, Schile, Berg, Schönberg, Webern, and Musil, just to mention a few well-known personalities. The great composer Brahms and his life-long friend Billroth, the great surgeon, had died only 4 years before.

Landsteiner's discovery remained in oblivion for a long time, until somebody read his work and applied it to blood transfusion. In 1916, Reuben Ottenberg at the Mount Sinai Hospital in New York, using blood grouping as proposed by Landsteiner and sodium citrate as the anticoagulant, successfully transfused 125 consecutive patients with zero mortality.

But what are the differences related to blood groups in detail? There are branched sugar structures hooked up to the proteins of the surface membrane of red blood cells. Slight differences in these sugars determine the different blood groups (Table 14.1). Anoter important issue is that there are different frequencies of the blood groups in different ethnic groups (Table 14.2). The blood groups are mainly associated with the red blood cells but they can also be found on other cells in the body, including white blood cells (WBCs), platelets, and other tissue cells. Additionally, soluble forms of ABO antigens are found in bodily fluids like saliva (in "secretors").

A further obstacle to transfusion was found to be due to the presence of natural antibodies (IgM type) in the blood with specificity for the particular sugar that is not present: individuals with blood group A have antibodies against B, those with group B have antibodies against A and those with group O have antibodies against both A and B, whilst those of group AB have neither of them. These antibodies to A and B antigens appear from birth and increase up until the age of 5, when they settle at adult levels. Why these natural antibodies are present is currently unknown but has interested hematologists and immunologists for many years. Transfusions among individuals of different blood groups (incompatible transfusion) cause reactions that can be fatal due to the massive destruction of the transfused RBCs and liberation of hemoglobin that precipitates in the kidney. Thus, those individuals with group O are known as Universal Donors, while those of group AB are known Universal Recipients.

As already described, for some years transfusions remained limited to the use of donors with blood group O—the universal donors. This severely limited the use of blood because donors with this group represent only 30 to 50% of the general population (except for a few Latin-American countries where the frequency is significantly higher).

For practical reasons, Landsteiner's group 0 (zero) is now identified with the letter 'O'.

In 1937, in collaboration with Alexander Wiener, Landsteiner identified another blood group system, which was called Rhesus (Rh, common to the Rhesus macaque monkeys). The chemical nature of this system is different from the ABO system as it made up of proteins, not sugars. Rhesus D is present in 85% of individuals but with a wide variation between different populations. In 1939, Levine highlighted the importance of this system by demonstrating that the Hemolytic Disease of Newborn*, occurred when an Rhesus D-negative mother (previously sensitised to D antigen by carrying a D-positive fetus) carries again a Rhesus -positive fetus in subsequent pregnancies. Nowadays, this condition has been almost eradicated by

Table 14.1 The three alleles model as proposed by Bernstein (1924)

		ABO Alleles inherited from the mother		
		A	B	O
ABO alleles inherited from the father	A	A	AB	A
	B	AB	B	B
	O	A	B	O
		Blood group of the offspring		

Table 14.2 Frequency of blood groups in the three main ethnic groups

	O (%)	A (%)	B (%)	AB (%)
Caucasian	44	43	9	4
African	49	27	20	4
Asian	43	27	25	5

using a specific prophylaxis* that prevents the primary immune response to antigen D— a vaccine administered in the third trimester of pregnancy and after the delivery. Therefore, the determination of Rh grouping is of major importance in women during the fertile period.

Another advance in transfusion therapy was the introduction of the Coombs Test, named after the scientist who proposed it. This test revealed the presence of antibodies in the serum or attached to the red cell surface. Robin Coombs proposed this test in 1945 and today it still represents one of the pillars for the 'definition' of blood compatibility and the study of the Immune Hemolytic Anemias. These immune disorders are due to the destruction of red cells by antibodies (Chap. 10). In further studies, thanks to the Coombs test, other minor systems causing transfusion reactions have been discovered. With the tests performed before a blood transfusion (cross-matching), it is now possible to prevent most, if not all, transfusion reactions. Moreover, today, there are automatic systems that allow the 'typing' of red cells and the recognition of antibodies that improve the safety of transfusion practice.

One more obstacle to transfusion was the frequent bacterial contamination of the containers used to collect blood. At the end of the nineteenth century, Pasteur and Koch demonstrated that numerous diseases were caused by bacteria. Joseph Lister, a surgeon from Edinburgh started using carbolic acid as a disinfectant for wounds and surgical injuries, to avoid infectious complications which, in the case of the lower limbs, often led to amputations. Lister called this method Anti-sepsis*. At the end of the nineteenth century, the Good Year Tire Company marketed the first latex gloves, which proved to be fundamentally important for maintaining antiseptic conditions during surgery. Finally, Charles Chamberland, a microbiologist and Pasteur Institute student proposed using an autoclave to sterilize surgical instruments and bottles for blood transfusion: bacteria and viruses are killed at a temperature of 121 °C.

Transfusion benefitted a great deal from these discoveries in the field of surgery and became safer thanks to the sterilization of blood containers and blood infusion sets. The introduction of plastic blood bags further facilitated blood donations and blood transfusion.

The use of blood typing became a major advance in criminology. In 1915 Leone Lattes, Professor of Legal Medicine and Criminal Anthropology (and only 14 years after the discovery of Landsteiner), developed methods to help identify individuals through their blood groups. To do this he proposed appropriate chemicals to extract blood from the blood stains detected at a crime scene.

Today, DNA technology has improved to the extent that with a few nanograms of tissue or blood, it is possible to distinguish an individual with a 99.9% certainty.

Chapter 15
Blood-Borne Viruses

During the war in Korea (1950–53), the prevalence of hepatitis amongst the American soldiers who received plasma was up to 20%, higher than those who received blood from voluntary donors. It was clear that the plasma processing methods based on pools made from thousands of donors were associated with a higher risk of hepatitis infection and that only one infected donation was sufficient to make the entire pool infectious. However, there were no tests to detect the agent (or the agents) causing hepatitis. Only much later was it discovered that hepatitis could be caused by at least three different viruses: A, B, and C. A few small British, French, and Italian pharmaceutical companies tried to solve the problem by using national plasma, but with little success, as hepatitis viruses were already widespread.

From the early 1960s, the hepatitis issue was clearly on the table, but nobody knew how to cope with it until 1965. At that time Blumberg in Australia identified a viral marker (a piece of hepatitis B virus molecule) present with a certain frequency in the blood of Australian Aborigines which he called 'Australia Antigen'. This marker was also found in hemophiliacs treated with plasma concentrates. Blumberg demonstrated that individuals with hemophilia were unfortunate victims because the plasma pools for the preparation of factor VIII concentrates were made up of very high numbers of donations. Hence, the hemophilia population progressively became infected with the hepatitis virus. In addition, a few of them had also been infected with HIV.

The HIV disease that frightened homosexuals was causing increasingly frequent deaths in their communities.

Blumberg's discovery opened the doors to the development of new donor screening methods. Until then, blood donors underwent screenings limited to syphilis and malaria. From 1970, the new tests for hepatitis B reduced the incidence of infection from 20%–25% to less than 10%. A further strong reduction of any type of infection was achieved with the exclusion of donors at high risk for AIDS (sexually promiscuous, drug-addicted, homosexuals). With the introduction of the HIV test in 1985, the risk of infection was reduced to less than 5%. However, it was only with the

G. Mariani et al., *Blood: The Science, History, and Mysteries of Life's Vital Flow*, https://doi.org/10.1007/978-3-031-92481-1_15

discovery of the hepatitis C virus in 1989 and the introduction of specific screening tests for this virus that the risk went down to less than 1%. It is important to note that performing more than one test was shown to reduce the residual risk. What matters is that each test has been improved over time in terms of precision and sensitivity. No doubt that an accurate selection of donors has contributed to a further lowering of the risk, now very close to zero.

Hepatitis A virus, being a virus transmitted almost exclusively by food, does not represent a problem for blood donation unless the donor is in the window period (the period that goes from infection to the disappearance of the virus from blood). There's no doubt that an accurate selection of donors is as important for blood donors as it is for plasma donors. As a consequence, the pharma industry policy concerning the procurement of plasma has radically changed to follow national and international regulations.

The impact of HIV was devastating, with many reports of hemophilia patients receiving infected plasma starting as early as the 1970s, from immigrants from Haiti, and drug addicts. What did these communities have in common? Nothing, it seemed. The media called it the 4H disease: homosexuals, hemophiliacs, Haitians, and heroin users. Subsequently, it was shown that HIV could be transmitted through blood, blood-derived products, and sex, but also by sharing syringes. Why did the inhabitants of Haiti have an increased risk? It was later discovered that in Haiti, the disease had a high incidence due to the socioeconomic situation of the Country, one of the poorest in the world and the sexual promiscuity.

Since the plasma market was global, the HIV epidemics reached Europe, Africa, and Asia. In Europe, AIDS cases in hemophiliacs became more and more frequent, but no solution was seen, nor was it possible to ban the concentrates. In retrospect, this would have been of little help because, it was later discovered, that AIDS in individuals with hemophilia has a very long incubation period, averaging around 9 years. Thus, the disaster had already occurred!

The number of hemophiliacs that became infected was variable depending on the country and the average amount of concentrates used in the different countries.

In March 1983, the American firm that had originally produced the first factor VIII concentrate marketed the first factor VIII treated with high temperatures, a method able to destroy the virus. Following this discovery, within 1 year a test for HIV screening became available, and its use became widespread and mandatory at the end of 1985. Currently, recombinant factors, free from any risk of viral contamination, account for greater than 70% of the market, a figure rapidly increasing.

Chapter 16
Blood Tumors and Their Therapies

Tumors are masses of cells where abnormal growth is caused by excessive division or delayed death. Cells in tumors are 'clonal', that is are derived from the same cell sharing the same genetic pattern.

Tumors of the blood are derived from the cells originating from the bone marrow—those involved in hematopoiesis.

The main blood tumors are shown in Table 16.1.

During tumor progression, secondary or tertiary somatic mutations may arise from the original clone, an event that complicates the course of the disease and can make it resistant to the therapies.

There are currently four main forms of therapy for blood tumors: chemotherapy, targeted therapy, immunotherapy, and stem cell therapy.

Chemotherapy

This term was initially proposed by Paul Ehrlich (1910) though his research was focused on infectious diseases, particularly syphilis, which, at that time, was a widespread infection. The compounds he employed were Salvarsan and Neo-Salvarsan, that were widely used in the treatment of syphilis until the advent of penicillin.

The use of chemotherapy in cancer treatment originated from the observation that mustard gas was very toxic to the bone marrow (causing myelosuppression*) and the lymphatic system, and so analogs of this compound were tested with some success in patients with lymphomas. Mustard gas is also called Yprite, deriving from the Belgian town Ypres where it was used in shells and bombs by the German army during WW1. The second antitumor drug to be developed was Methotrexate, an antagonist of vitamin B9 (folic acid), which made it possible, for the first time, to treat childhood acute leukemia with some success.

© The Author(s), under exclusive license to Springer Nature Switzerland AG 2025   97
G. Mariani et al., *Blood: The Science, History, and Mysteries of Life's Vital Flow*, https://doi.org/10.1007/978-3-031-92481-1_16

Table 16.1 Classification of the blood tumors: some appear malignant from the very beginning, while others are considered to be pre-neoplastic since they may evolve later to malignant disorders. Malignant blood tumors arise from mutations occurring in the bone marrow precursors or the stem cells. Mutations can be various, and even within a given tumor, clinical differences are seen

Malignant Tumors	Lymphomas	Hodgkin (Hodgkin Disease, HD) Non-Hodgkin Lymphoma
	Acute Leukemias	Myeloid (AML) Lymphoid (ALL) Monocytic Myelomonocytic
	Monoclonal gammopathies	Plasma-cell leukemia Multiple Myeloma (MM) Smoldering Myeloma
	Chronic Leukemias	Chronic Lymphocityc Leukemia (CLL) Chronic myeloid Leukemia (CML)
Pre-neoplastic syndromes	Myelodysplastic syndromes (MDS) > acute leukemias Monoclonal Gammopathies of uncertain significance > multiple myeloma	

By the end of the 1950s and 60s, other drugs were obtained from the Periwinkle plant (Catharanthus roseus) that grows in Madagascar. These Vinca Alkaloids (Vincristine and Vinblastine) were isolated from the leaves of this plant and were shown to be very active in treating a number of blood malignancies.

Chemotherapies have different mechanisms of action because they act on different phases of cell replication. DNA synthesis is necessary for cells to divide so that drugs that inhibit this important cell activity (methotrexate, 6-mercaptopurine, thioguanine, and other metabolites) are effective to prevent their replication. Alkylating agents are active in all phases of the cell cycle because they bind DNA and prevent its transcription. In contrast, anti-mitotic agents (such as Vinca alkaloids) act during the final stages of the cell cycle, preventing the formation of the chromosomal spindle and, therefore, blocking cell mitosis.

As soon as other products were obtained or synthesized, combinations of drugs with different mechanisms of action, and standard doses and in various sequences were tested in 'Therapeutic Protocols'. Combinations of drugs were shown to be more efficacious than the drugs used alone. Firstly, this approach was empirically used in patients (in vivo), but by the 1970s and 80 s, antitumor drugs were tested using cells that could be grown outside the body in special media and in tissue cultures (in vitro): cell death, cell senescence, apoptosis*, and nuclear abnormalities could be measured and analyzed on living cells. Although there is not always a direct correspondence between the in vitro and the in vivo efficacy, these methods have largely been used by the pharmaceutical industry to standardize drug efficacy. However, the final assessment of drug efficacy is based on controlled studies—clinical trials (validated by statistical methods) approved by special committees (ethical committees) and subsequently after a period of post-marketing drug surveillance. The goal of chemotherapy is to destroy as many tumoral cells as possible, leaving a number of normal stem cells alive sufficient to reproduce a normal marrow. This achievement is called 'Minimal Residual Disease'* since it is postulated that some, unseen, malignant cells remain. Clinical trials can last years before a drug is finally approved for general distribution.

Targeted Therapy

This type of therapy targets biochemical reactions in cancer cells that are important for their survival and activation. These include enzymes such as asparaginase and enzyme inhibitors such as imatinib or ibrutinib, effective for the management of specific types of leukemias.

Immunotherapy

Another very important step in treatment resulted with the introduction of Immunotherapy using Monoclonal Antibodies (MAB): these antibodies are identical to each other and are laboratori-produced in inducing. Many MABs are already in use to treat tumors of the blood (mainly Chronic Lymphoid leukemia, lymphomas and myeloma) and numerous (more than 100 or so are in the last phases of clinical trials for a variety of different types of cancer). MAB are used alone or in combination with chemotherapy. MAB as drugs are recognized by having 'mab' acronym at the end of the drug name e.g., rituximab, daratumumab etc. However, some only use the company drug name e.g. Herceptin. This is a MAB that targets a specific tumor protein present in a third of breast cancers.

It is now possible to arm the killer T cells (CD8 plated T cells) of a cancer patient with MABs that create, the CAR T cells able to reduce the tumor mass.

Stem Cell Therapy

You will remember that the hematologist Janet Vaughan studied the effects of radiation on bone marrow. It is also used to treat some solid tumors but causes mutations and strongly depresses the bone marrow activity. One of the most important findings of these studies on bone marrow has led to the implementation of Bone Marrow Transplantation. But how transplantation works?

Initially, the 'sick' marrow is eradicated either through lethal doses of irradiation and/or high-dose chemotherapy. After 2–3 days, to save the patient from the absence of blood production, normal stem cells (plated CD34) are transfused. Stem Cells reach the empty hematopoietic niches and slowly grow, giving rise to new hematopoiesis. The new marrow will start to produce normal blood cells within 2–4 weeks.

Let's imagine a wheat field infested with weeds and poppies: to be able to replant the field, the farmer must cut everything- the wheat, poppies, and weeds, burn the stubble—and, finally, plow and sow the ground again. This is what happens when a bone marrow transplant is carried out: only by destroying both the sick marrow (poppies and weeds) and the remaining healthy marrow (the wheat) is it possible to create the environment for normal hematopoiesis.

But how was this procedure originally thought? After years of experimental studies on animal models, in 1956, in Cooperstown, in the state of New York, Donall Thomas performed the first marrow transplant between identical twins: after the eradication of all the sick marrow cells with a lethal dose of gamma rays (ionizing radiation*) in the ill twin, he was transfused with the marrow of the healthy twin. Thomas demonstrated, for the first time, that the eradication of leukemia was possible through the complete reconstitution of a normal marrow. In 1990, he received the Nobel prize for his numerous studies on bone marrow biology and bone marrow transplantation.

However, the availability of an identical twin is a rare event (about 1/300 pregnancies), thus, the procedure would have had a very limited application because each individual exhibits specific proteins in his cells surface (called Human Leukocyte Antigens, HLA) that represent an obstacle to the colonization of the foreign cells. In fact, these are recognized as foreigners (non-self) causing a strong immunological reaction which is so-called Graft Versus Host Disease* that can be deadly. HLA was first discovered in white blood cells, but it is present in every cell of the body, a feature that makes each individual different from another. Only in identical twins are these proteins the same, as is the case of the blood groups! These MHC proteins are the main cause of transplant rejection (all transplants, not only those of the bone marrow) since the cells of the immune system attack and destroy those cells recognized as non-self.

Only with the discovery of HLA and the development of laboratory methods for their evaluation by Jean Dausset (1958–1968) became possible, by using 'compatible' marrows, to perform transplants between non-identical individuals: this procedure is called Allogeneic* (which means: different genes) transplant, The same occurs in the case of a transplant from a family member because HLA genes share a limited grade of similarity which is better in related individuals; in fact, there is a 1 in 4 chance that siblings share similar HLA antigen setting. Worldwide, approximately 45% of transplants are performed amongst related individuals, but this figure is expected to become lower due to the general reduction in family size.

To increase the chance of finding 'compatible marrow'* outside family members, national and international Registries have been created that gather the HLA types of numerous potential marrow donors (unrelated allogenic transplant): The American registry (National Marrow Donor Program) had more than 9 million donors in 2022. The UK, the Italian and the Polish registries include about 500,000 donors each, that are not enough for the needs of the countries. Indeed, the larger the registry, the higher the probability of finding a compatible donor: a recent study conducted in the USA showed that the probability of finding a compatible donor in the same ethnic group can be over 90%.

The success of a transplant is evaluated by assessing the number of donor marrow cells present after the procedure: if it is 100%, all the tumor cells have been destroyed. This result is termed Complete *Chimerism* (taken from Greek mythology: the chimera* was a monster with a body made up of different animals). Partial Chimerism, instead, is associated with a high risk of relapse. In the case of complete chimerism, the recipient changes the blood group to that of the donor (if different), but the DNA of the other tissues (liver, brain, skin, bowel, etc.) remains unchanged.

The use of bone marrow as a source of CD34-plated stem cells has now been superseded by taking the stem cells out of the peripheral blood of a donor. GCSF (Chap. 8)—a cytokine is given to the donor to 'drive' some of these stem cells from the bone marrow into the bloodstream, and these can be enriched using a machine called 'blood cell processor'. Stem Cells are subsequently transfused to the recipient who has been treated to remove all cancer cells by chemotherapy and or radiotherapy as described above.

Gene Therapy

More recently, a more sophisticated and curative approach for treating tumors has been proposed: Gene Therapy However, this procedure can be performed only in highly specialized medical facilities.

Gene Therapy is a technology based on the transfer of one (or more) genes to treat or prevent the damage caused by genetic disorders. Gene therapy is (within certain limits) less invasive and less risky compared to organ transplantation.

Essentially, the purpose of gene therapy is to correct a genetic defect that underlies a congenital disease. Gene therapy can be of two types: (1) Somatic gene therapy, where genes with a therapeutic function are inserted in a variety of cells except for gametes (oocytes, spermatozoa) and stem cells. (2) Germline gene therapy, where germline cells are modified through the introduction of modified genes into the gametes, a change that is inherited by the next generations. This type is currently not allowed by most health regulatory agencies mostly because of ethical issues.

In 1996, a group of hematologists in Milan headed by Dr. Aiuti, performed the first fully successful gene therapy approach using hematopoietic stem cells as vectors to treat ADA*-Severe-Combined-Immunodeficiency. One wonders how is it possible that the malfunction of a single enzyme can cause a disease that is lethal in children within the first year of life. This small enzyme has the function of eliminating deoxyadenosine, a substance that results from the destruction (or catabolism) of DNA. If this small enzyme does not work, the deoxy-adenosine accumulates in the cells and prevents DNA synthesis, leading to their death by apoptosis. Thus, very few T cells are available and their function is severely impaired. As a result, the function of their immune system is severely compromised. Children with this condition (called Bubble Boy disease) must be protected from contact with infectious agents, like in a bubble. The scientists from Milan inserted the gene of this enzyme into a retrovirus; this modified virus was used to infect stem cells extracted from the patient. Autologous* stem cells, then colonize the marrow and differentiate into myeloid and lymphoid progenitor cells. By 2021, 40 children had been treated with an average age of one and a half years, and half of them were alive, the longest survival being more than 13 years. All the children had various infectious complications in the initial period since time is required for the reconstitution of the immune system. One child developed acute leukemia but was successfully treated. There is no doubt that this experience was a great success, and the EMA* in 2016 registered the procedure. Other Gene Therapy approaches have been carried out in Hemophilia A and B with good results (cessation of hemorrhages) and in a type of Retina Dystrophy with improvement in the visual capacity. A very useful instrument for those who are interested in studying genetic disorders is the site called OMIM* (Online Mendelian Inheritance in Man), a catalog of human genes and genetic disorders continuously updated.

Gene therapy may be used to insert functional genes into the CD34 stem cells of children with faulty genes using the technique described above. Over 100 faulty genes are responsible for producing proteins important in the development of the immune system and its function. This therapy together with the gene editing technique (see below) is going to revolutionize the treatment of several blood disorders. However, a concern inherent with Gene therapy is that the insertion of a functional gene occurs randomly in the DNA of the patient and can create 'new genes' that might promote tumors. This side effect has been observed in some clinical trials.

Gene Editing

This amazing new technique called CRISPR-Cas9 has been shown to work like 'gene scissors'. It is used to directly remove the faulty gene and put in the functional gene. For developing this gene editing technology, the Nobel Prize in Chemistry in 2020 was awarded jointly to Emmanuelle Charpentier and Jennifer A. Doudna. Their work has been instrumental in allowing precise modifications to DNA Wide-ranging applications in science, medicine, and biotechnology are expected. The advantage of this technology over gene therapy is that the gene can be inserted more precisely into the DNA and not randomly. This technology has already been used to cure patients with sickle cell anemia. Stem cells from a patient with this hemolytic disease are taken, modified with the functional gene through the CRISPR technology, and returned to the patient.

This procedure is being used to test the potential of gene editing in other blood disorders, such as thalassemia.

Source of Figures

Fig. 2.1 Audrey Davis: Bloodletting Instruments in the National Museum of History & Technology, 1983 ISBN-10091549700X

Fig. 3.1 Anne Schraff: Dr. Charles Drew Blood Bank Innovator. Enslow Publishing, LLC, 2003

We are http://rubriche.eusebiano.it/wp-content/uploads/sites/3/2015/10/circolazione-galenosm.jpg?x59481

Drawing and Annotations by Leonardo—1510 circa—Collection Windsor Castle, United Kingdom. Royal Collection Trust/© Her Majesty Queen Elizabeth II 2018

https://microbiologyinfo.com/blood-cells-types-functions/. Last updated: August 10, 2022 by Sagar Aryal https://it.wikipedia.org/wiki/Norman_Bethune

Note

We would like to thank Rita Peralta M.D., PhD for her translation of the text from an early Italian version.

Glossary

Acquired immunity   One of the two main types of immunity in vertebrates (the other being the innate immune system). Synonymous: adaptive immunity

ADA-deaminase   Enzyme involved in purine metabolism. It is needed for the breakdown of adenosine from food and for the turnover of nucleic acids in tissues.

Allogeneic bone marrow transplant   When healthy stem cells from a donor are used to replace bone marrow that is not producing enough blood cells

Antibody   Antibodies are large, Y-shaped proteins belonging to the immunoglobulin superfamily which are used by the immune system to identify and neutralize bacteria, viruses, fungi and parasites. Synonyms: immunoglobulins (Ig)

Antigen   A small part of a microorganism or a cell (both have many antigens) that antibody attaches to; also recognised by T cell and B cell receptors (sensors).

Antisepsis   The practice of *using anti-bacterial, anti-viral, and anti-fungal substances on living skin, tissue or devices* to prevent spread of infections.

Apoptosis   A form of programmed cell death that occurs in cells of multicellular organisms. To be distinguished from Necrosis (unprogrammed cell death).

Autologous bone marrow transplantation   A procedure in which a patient's healthy stem cells are collected from the blood or bone marrow before treatment, stored, and then given back to the patient after myelosuppression.

Bloodletting   Drawing blood from an individual to prevent or treat disease.

Bone Marrow Niche   The bone marrow niche is an environment made up of cells including osteoblasts, osteoclasts, adipocytes and stromal cells. Depending on the microenvironment, the Stem Cells develop into specific mature blood cells i.e. Monocytes, red blood cells etc.

CD cluster determinant   The cluster determinant or cluster of differentiation is a protocol used for the identification and investigation of cell surface and cytoplasmic molecules, that are used as targets for cell immunophenotyping. Synonym: cluster of differentiation o cluster of designation

Cellular immunity   Cellular immunity, also known as cell-mediated immunity, is an immune system based on the activation of phagocytes, T-cytotoxic cells and the release of cytokines.

Chemotherapy   Chemotherapy is a treatment method that utilizes a standard regimen of one or more anti-cancer drugs in association.

Chimera/Chimerism   In genetics, the term chimera applies to organs/organisms composed of cells from different individuals/genotypes. Examples include bone marrow or organ transplant recipients.

Clone, cellular clone   A *clone* is a group of identical cells sharing a common ancestry and sharing the same genotype

Compatible Marrow   Marrow from a healthy donor who has human leukocyte antigens (HLA) as similar to the recipient's as possible

Cytokines   A broad category of small hormone-like proteins important in cell signalling. Synonymous: Growth Factors, Chemokines, Lymphokines

Cytoplasm   A gelatinous fluid that fills the interior of the cells, made up of water, salts and a number of molecules.

DNA   Deoxyribonucleic acid (DNA) is the molecule that carries genetic information for the development and functioning of an organism. DNA is made up of two linked strands that wind around each other to resemble a twisted ladder, a shape known as a double helix. Each strand has a backbone made of alternating sugar (deoxyribose) and phosphate groups. Attached to each sugar is one of following bases: adenine (A), cytosine (C), guanine (G) or thymine (T).

Double Helix   Double helix is a term used to describe the physical structure of DNA

EMA   EMA guarantees the scientific evaluation, supervision & safety monitoring of human & veterinary medicines in the EU

Epitope   Also known as antigenic determinant, is the part of an antigen recognized by the immune system. Synonymous: antigenic determinant

Erythrocytes   Term used in academia and medical publishing to identify the red blood cells

Exchange-transfusion   Medical procedure to replace patient's blood with donor blood

FDA   Food and Drug Administration guarantees the scientific evaluation, supervision & safety monitoring of human & veterinary medicines in the USA

Flow cytometry (FC)   A technique used to identify and measure the physical and chemical characteristics of cells or particles in a fluid moiety. See cluster determinants

Graft Versus Host Disease (GVHD)   Graft versus Host Disease (GvHD) is the immune reaction exerted by transplanted cells (from the donor) against the tissues of the person receiving them (recipient).

Growth Factors   See Cytokines

Hemolytic Disease of the Newborn   Hemolytic disease of the newborn is a blood disorder that results from mismatch of Rhesus D antigen between the mother and her baby.

Humoral Immunity Is the type of immunity that is mediated by antibodies including complement proteins, and certain antimicrobial peptides—located in extracellular fluids. Synonym: antibody-mediated immunity

Immunophenotype The immunochemical and immunohistochemical features of a cell or group of cells identifiable by flow-cytometry

Immunotherapy Immunotherapy is a type of cancer treatment that fight disease using components of the immune system. Also used to treat other diseases including autoimmunity etc.

Infection A disease caused by bacteria, viruses, fungi and parasites

Innate/Natural Immunity The first line of defence against invading pathogens. Synonymous: natural immunity

Ionizing radiations A form of radiation with the potential of damaging living cells by breaking their molecular bonds and displacing electrons

Lyophilization Lyophilization is a water removal process used to preserve perishable materials, to extend their shelf life and making them more convenient for transport.

Lysis The breakdown of a cell caused by damage to its membrane

Macrophage A white blood cell that eats microorganisms, eliminates dead cells, and stimulates other immune system cells through cytokines

Menorrhagia It refers to menstrual bleeding lasting longer than 7 days or bleeding occurring for a longer time than that typical for a given individual. Synonym: heavy menstrual bleeding

Metabolic Syndrome A common clinical issue characterized by overweight, high blood pressure, hyperlipidemia, and reduced tolerance to sugars (prediabetes).

Metrorrhagia It refers to bleeding occurring during the intermenstrual period. Also called intermenstrual bleeding,

Micronutrients Chemical elements or substances required in trace amounts for the optimal growth and development of living organisms as opposed to Macronutrients that are nutrietns needed in large amounts as carbohydrates, proteins, and fats.

Microphage Microphages are small phagocytes, especially neutrophils and eosinophils.

Minimal Residual Disease (MRD) Minimal residual disease is *a small (or the smallest) number of cancer cells left in the body after treatment.*

Mucosa The skin that surrounds the inner surface of body parts, like the nose and mouth, and creates mucus to shield them.

Myelosuppression Decrease in the ability of the bone marrow to produce blood cells. Myelosuppression may occur when the stem cells are damaged (such as by chemotherapy drugs), or when it is crowded (by tumor cells or fibrosis).

Natural Killer cells Blood cells that respond quickly to a wide variety of pathological challenges.

Necrosis A form of cell injury which result in the premature death of cells by autolysis.

Nucleus The cellular organelle that contains the chromosomes.

OMIM   OMIM (Online Mendelian Inheritance in Man) is a catalog of human genes and genetic disorders, with links to literature references, sequence records, maps, and related databases. It is based on the book, Mendelian Inheritance in Man.

Phenotype   Phenotype refers to an individual's traits, such as height, eye color and blood type as we can observe them. A person's phenotype is determined by both his genomic makeup (genotype) and environmental factors.

Phlebotomy   Synonym of bloodletting.

Plethora/Plethoric   A condition characterized by excess of blood in the circulation and a reddish complexion.

Prophylaxis   The practice of taking measures to prevent a disease.

Receptor   Chemical structures, composed of protein and/or sugars, that receive and transduce signals inside the cell

Ribosomes   Very small yet very important organelles essential for the process called translation important to make proteins

RNA   Ribonucleic acid (abbreviated RNA) is a nucleic acid present in living cells that has structural similarities to DNA. Unlike DNA, however, RNA is most often single-stranded. An RNA molecule has a backbone made of alternating phosphate groups and the sugar ribose, rather than the deoxyribose found in DNA. Attached to each sugar is one of four bases: adenine (A), uracil (U), cytosine (C) or guanine (G).

Stem cells   Stem cells are a special type of cell with two important attributes. They can reproduce themselves, that is, they renew themselves, and they can give rise to other cells in a process known as differentiation.

References

Principal References

Hayes, B. (2006). *Five quarts. A personal and natural history of blood*. Random House.
Hoffman, R., et al. (2017). *Hematology. Basic principles and practice* (7th ed.). Elsevier.
Kean, S. (2012). *The violinist's thumb*. Back Bay Books/Little, Brown and Co.
Starr, D. (2002). *Blood. An epic history of medicine and commerce*. Harper Perennial.
Tucker, H. (2012). *Blood work. A tale of medicine & murder in the scientific revolution*. Norton & Company.

Other References

Bordignon, C. (2017). Twenty-five years of gene therapy for genetic disease and leukemia: The road to marketing authorization of the first *ex vivo* gene therapies. *Journal of Autoimmunity, 85*, 98–102.
Canellos, G. P. (2014). Treatment of Hodgkin lymphoma: A 50-year perspective. *Journal of Clinical Oncology, 3*, 163–168.
Chabner, B. A., & Roberts, T. G. (2005). Timeline: Chemotherapy and the war on cancer. *Nature Reviews Cancer, 5*, 65–72.
Cicalese, M. P., et al. (2018). Gene therapy for adenosine deaminase deficiency: A comprehensive evaluation of short- and medium-term safety. *Molecular Therapy, 26*, 917–931.
Delioux de Savignac, J. (1861). *Principes de la Doctrine e de la méthose en médicine*. Victor Masson et Fils.
Figes, O. (2017). *A people's tragedy. The Russian Revolution*. Penguin-Random House.
Gragert, L., et al. (2014). HLA match likelihood for hematopoietic stem-cell graft in the US registry. *The New England Journal of Medicine, 371*, 339–348.
Leslie e altri. (1997). History of post-transfusion hepatitis. *Clinical Chemistry, 43*, 1487–1493.
Martelli, M. F., et al. (2014). HLA-haploidentical transplantation with regulatory and consentional T-cell adoptive immunotherapy prevents acute leukemia relapse. *Blood, 124*, 638–644.
McLean, E., et al. (2009). Worldwide prevalence of anaemia. WHO Vitamin and Mineral Nutrition Information System, 1993–2005. *Public Health Nutrition, 12*, 444–454.

Meletis, J., & Kostantinpoulos, K. (2010). The beliefs, myths and reality surrounding the word hema (blood) from homer to the present. *Anemia, 2010*, 857657.

Metcalf, D. (2008). Hematopoietic cytokines. *Blood, 111*, 485–491.

Nathwani, A. C., et al. (2017). Advances in gene therapy for hemophilia. *Human Gene Therapy, 28*, 1004–1012.

Niederwieser, D., et al. (2016). Hematopoietic stem cell transplantation activity worldwide in 2012 and a SWOT analysis of the Worldwide Network for Blood and Marrow Transplantation Group (WBMT) including the global survey. *Bone Marrow Transplantation, 51*, 778–785.

Parapia, L. A. (2008). History of bloodletting by phlebotomy. *British Journal of Haematology, 143*, 490–495.

Remuzzi, G. (2012). Ethical disputes still beset Italian medicine 150 after Count Cavour's death. *Lancet, 379*, 1068–1073.

Silva, A. S., et al. (2011). A multiscale model of the bone marrow and hematopoiesis. *Mathematical Biosciences and Engineering, 8*, 643–658.

GPSR Compliance
The European Union's (EU) General Product Safety Regulation (GPSR) is a set
of rules that requires consumer products to be safe and our obligations to
ensure this.

If you have any concerns about our products, you can contact us on

ProductSafety@springernature.com

In case Publisher is established outside the EU, the EU authorized
representative is:

Springer Nature Customer Service Center GmbH
Europaplatz 3
69115 Heidelberg, Germany